SJÖGREN'S SYNDROME: AN ANTI-INFLAMMATORY COOKBOOK FOR AUTOIMMUNE DISORDER

Boost Your Immunity and Health with High Fiber, Nutritious Recipes to Prevent Symptoms and Promote Wellness

Daria Cross, MD

COPYRIGHT PAGE

The information in this book is not intended, under any circumstances, to replace or serve as a substitute for professional medical advice, diagnosis, or treatment. Any individual seeking advice regarding a medical condition or seeking treatment options should always consult with a qualified healthcare provider or physician. The author and publisher explicitly disclaim any responsibility for adverse effects or consequences arising from the utilization of the recipes or information presented in this cookbook.

Table of Contents

PART 1: UNDERSTANDING SJÖGREN'S SYNDROME AND INFLAMMATION

Sjogren's syndrome is an autoimmune disease that causes your immune system to go haywire and attack healthy cells instead of invading bacteria or viruses. Your white blood cells, which normally protect you from germs, attack the glands that are in charge of making moisture. When that happens, the glands can't produce tears and saliva, so your eyes, mouth, and other parts of your body dry out.

As a systemic disease, affecting the entire body, symptoms may remain steady or worsen overtime. There is no one single progression of the disease and this can make it challenging for patients and their physicians. While some people experience mild discomfort, others suffer debilitating symptoms that greatly impair their functioning. Early diagnosis and proper treatments are important as they may prevent serious complications and greatly improve a patient's quality of life.

About half of the time Sjögren's occurs alone, and the other half it occurs in the presence of another autoimmune connective tissue disease such as Rheumatoid Arthritis, Lupus, or Scleroderma.

In addition, Sjögren's is often misrepresented as a rare disease, however it is estimated that there are four million Americans living with this disease, making it one of the most prevalent autoimmune diseases.

Sjögren's syndrome is a long-lasting disorder that affects females more often than men. It is often diagnosed in females during middle age or after menopause, but it can affect anyone at any age (including children).

Currently, there is no cure for Sjögren's syndrome. Treatment may include drugs to reduce the effect on the immune system and relieve other symptoms.

Sjogren's syndrome Types

You might hear your doctor talk about a couple of types of Sjogren's disease:

Primary Sjogren's syndrome: This means you have it without any other autoimmune rheumatic disease.

Secondary Sjogren's syndrome: This term is used to describe Sjogren's that occurs along with another autoimmune or rheumatic disease, such as rheumatoid arthritis, scleroderma, or lupus.

Symptoms and Diagnosis

The main symptoms of Sjögren's syndrome are dry eyes and a dry mouth, but it can also cause several other problems.

Each person is affected differently. For some people the condition may just be a bit of a nuisance, while for others it can have a big impact on their daily life.

There are many conditions that can cause similar symptoms. See a GP if you have any symptoms you're worried about.

Dry eyes

Signs that you may have dry eyes include:

Burning, stinging or itchy eyes

A feeling of grit or sand in your eyes

Sore, red and swollen eyelids

Discomfort when looking at lights

Sticky eyelids when you wake up

Blurred vision

These symptoms may be worse when the air is dry, for example, when you're somewhere that's windy, smoky or air conditioned.

Dry eyes can be caused by many conditions besides Sjögren's syndrome.

Read more about dry eyes.

Dry mouth

Signs that you may have a dry mouth include:

Feeling like food gets stuck in your mouth or throat, especially dry foods like crackers

Needing to drink water while you're eating to help you swallow food

Your tongue sticking to the roof of your mouth

A hoarse voice

A smooth, red tongue

A change in how food tastes

Dry, sore and cracked skin at the corners of your lips

Problems such as tooth decay, gum disease, mouth ulcers, and oral thrush (a fungal infection that can cause a raw, red or white tongue)

Other reasons for a dry mouth include things such as diabetes or medicines.

Read more about a dry mouth.

Other symptoms

Other possible symptoms of Sjögren's syndrome can include:

Dry, itchy skin

Severe tiredness and exhaustion

Vaginal dryness in women, which can make sex painful

Rashes (especially after being in the sun)

A dry cough that does not go away

Swelling between the jaw and ears (swollen salivary glands)

Muscle pain

Joint pain, stiffness and swelling

Difficulty with concentrating, remembering, and reasoning

Some people with Sjögren's syndrome also have other, closely linked conditions, such as Raynaud's phenomenon (a condition that affects blood supply to your fingers and toes).

Diagnosis

See a GP if you have symptoms of Sjögren's syndrome.

They'll ask about your symptoms and look at your eyes and mouth to check for any obvious problems.

Because there are many conditions with similar symptoms to Sjögren's syndrome, it can be very difficult for a GP to diagnose.

They can refer you to a specialist for further checks, if needed.

Blood tests

Blood tests can be done to look for antibodies in your blood. Antibodies are substances produced by your immune system (the body's defence against infection) to attack germs.

In Sjögren's syndrome, the immune system produces antibodies that attack healthy areas of the body. These can be found during a blood test.

But not everyone with Sjögren's syndrome has these antibodies, so you may have the condition even if a blood test does not find them.

Checking the layer of tears on your eyes

An eye doctor (ophthalmologist) may do a test to look at the layer of tears that forms across the front of your eyes.

Harmless coloured drops are put in your eyes to make the layer of tears easier to see for a short time. A special microscope with a light is then used to look at your eyes.

If the layer of tears is very patchy, it could be a sign of Sjögren's syndrome.

Testing a piece of lip tissue

In people with Sjögren's syndrome, clumps of white blood cells, which are produced by the immune system, can form inside the cells where spit (saliva) is produced.

To check for this, a very small piece of tissue from the inside of your lip may be removed and looked at under a microscope. This is known as a lip biopsy.

Local anaesthetic is injected into your lip to numb it before the procedure.

Other tests

Occasionally, other tests may be done. These may include:

A spit test – you spit as much saliva as you can into a cup over a 5-minute period and the amount is then measured or weighed

Measuring how many tears you produce – small strips of paper are placed in your lower eyelid for 5 minutes to see how much of the paper is soaked with tears

Producing less saliva or fewer tears than normal can be a sign of Sjögren's syndrome.

Causes and Risk Factors

What causes Sjögren's syndrome?

Sjögren's syndrome is an autoimmune disease. Autoimmune diseases happen when your immune system mistakenly damages your body instead of protecting it. Experts aren't sure what makes your immune system attack your glands and cause Sjögren's syndrome.

Primary Sjögren's syndrome happens with no known trigger or cause.

Other health conditions trigger secondary Sjögren's syndrome, especially other autoimmune diseases and some viral infections.

Viral infections that can trigger secondary Sjögren's syndrome include:

Hepatitis C.

Cytomegalovirus (CMV).

Epstein-Barr virus.

Human T-lymphotropic virus 1 (HTLV).

COVID-19.

Any autoimmune disease can trigger secondary Sjögren's syndrome. Some autoimmune diseases that are related to Sjögren's syndrome include:

Rheumatoid arthritis.

Psoriatic arthritis.

Lupus

Even though studies have linked Sjögren's syndrome to other conditions, there's no guarantee you'll develop it if you have these conditions.

Similarly, Sjögren's syndrome might make you more likely to develop other autoimmune conditions, but that doesn't mean you definitely will.

What are the risk factors for Sjögren's syndrome?

Anyone can develop Sjögren's syndrome, but certain groups of people are more likely to have it:

Women and people assigned female at birth (AFAB): More than 90% of people with Sjögren's syndrome are AFAB. People assigned male at birth (AMAB) can develop it, but it's much less common.

People with other autoimmune diseases: Around half of people with Sjögren's syndrome have at least one other autoimmune condition.

People between the ages of 45 and 55: Children, younger adults and adults older than 55 can have Sjögren's syndrome, but it usually develops in adults in that age range.

People who have a biological relative with Sjögren's syndrome: Around 10% of people with Sjögren's syndrome have a direct relative (a biological parent or sibling) with it, too.

Complications

Sjögren's syndrome can sometimes lead to further problems, or you may have it alongside other conditions.

Eye problems

If you have very dry eyes and they're not treated, there's a risk the front layer of your eyes could become damaged over time. This could lead to permanent vision problems.

There are several treatments for dry eyes that can help reduce this risk. Read about them on our page about treatment for Sjögren's syndrome. You should also have regular check-ups with an optician so any problems are found early.

Contact a GP as soon as possible if you have problems with your vision.

Find an optician

Lung problems

Sjögren's syndrome can sometimes affect the lungs and cause problems such as:

Lung infections

Widening of the airways in the lungs (bronchiectasis)

Scarring of the lungs

If you smoke, quitting may help reduce the risk of these conditions. Read more about stopping smoking.

See a GP if you have a cough, wheezing or shortness of breath that does not go away.

Pregnancy complications

Most women with Sjögren's syndrome can get pregnant and have healthy babies.

But if you're planning a pregnancy, it's a good idea to get advice from a GP or specialist because there's a small risk of complications for some women.

These include:

A rash on the baby that lasts a few weeks

Serious heart problems in the baby

These problems can happen if you have certain antibodies (produced by your immune system) sometimes found in people with Sjögren's syndrome. A blood test can be done to look for these.

If these antibodies are found, you can still get pregnant, but you may need extra care from a specialist during your pregnancy and after the birth.

Cancer

People with Sjögren's syndrome have an increased risk of getting a type of cancer called non-Hodgkin lymphoma.

This affects the lymphatic system, a network of vessels and glands found throughout the body.

Research shows people with Sjögren's syndrome are about 5 times more likely to get non-Hodgkin lymphoma than people who do not have the condition. But the chances of getting it are still small.

See a GP if you have symptoms of non-Hodgkin lymphoma, such as:

Painless swollen glands, usually in your neck, armpit or groin

Night sweats

Unintended weight loss

Non-Hodgkin lymphoma can often be cured if it's found early.

Other problems

Other conditions that have been linked to Sjögren's syndrome include:

Raynaud's phenomenon – restricted blood flow to the hands and feet, which can cause them to feel cold, numb and painful

An underactive thyroid gland (hypothyroidism) – which can cause tiredness and weight gain

Irritable bowel syndrome (IBS) – which can cause tummy pain, diarrhoea or constipation

Peripheral neuropathy – a condition that causes loss of feeling in the hands and feet

Kidney problems – such as kidney inflammation or kidney stones

Inflammation of the blood vessels (Sjogren's syndrome) – which can cause a rash that looks like small bruises or reddish-purple spots

Treatment Strategies

A Sjögren's patient's treatment path should be decided on a case-by-case basis after the potential benefits and side-effects are weighed by patients and their healthcare providers. Since Sjögren's affects each patient differently, a personalized plan should be developed by you and your physician, dentist, eye care provider and other specialists about how to treat your various symptoms.

In some cases, lifestyle changes can help certain symptoms such as fatigue and gastro-intestinal reflux, and over-the-counter products can help alleviate symptoms such as dryness. Sjögren's patients are often managed with a combination of management strategies, over-the-counter products and prescription drugs. Most patients will need prescription medications at some point in their disease course to help control their disease and reduce the potential for complications.

A number of different medications are available that can be used to manage symptoms. Currently, no single medication has been conclusively proven to slow the progression of Sjögren's or treat all aspects of the disease.

Prescription Treatments

Below are a few of the prescription treatments available, but by no means is this an exhaustive list. Talk to your physician for more information.

Non-Steroidal Anti-Inflammatory Drugs (NSAIDs)

NSAIDs are often a first-line therapy used in Sjögren's and reduce inflammation which is often high in Sjögren's. NSAIDs reduce the production of prostaglandins that promote inflammation and pain. NSAIDs include common over-the-counter medications such as aspirin, ibuprofen (Advil, Motrin) and naproxen (Aleve), but many prescription NSAID drugs are available. The most common side effect of NSAIDs is stomach upset, and, rarely, NSAIDs might cause stomach or gastrointestinal bleeding or ulceration. One class of NSAIDs, cox-2 inhibitors, is less likely to cause stomach problems but may have different potential side effects that should be discussed with your doctor.

Corticosteroids

Corticosteroids, a class of drugs that includes prednisone, are fast-acting and may be highly successful in halting severe symptoms of Sjögren's and/or a flare. Short-term use (up to one month) might be sufficient before tapering off completely, but sometimes long-term use (more than one month) is necessary. If a patient is prescribed corticosteroids for long-term use, the patient will start at a higher dose and taper down to a lower, maintenance dose. Corticosteroids have many potential side effects ranging from minor to more severe, so physicians may try to find a steroid-sparing drug that reduces a patient's symptoms if a patient is on corticosteroids for a long period.

Disease-Modifying Anti Rheumatic Drugs (DMARDs)

DMARDs modify the way the immune system functions, so instead of simply treating symptoms, DMARDs regulate abnormal immune responses. Unlike corticosteroids, these drugs do not produce an immediate effect but take time to have an impact on symptoms and before a patient feels a difference.

Hydroxychloroquine (Plaquenil®)

The most commonly prescribed DMARD is hydroxychloroquine (Plaquenil®). It is often prescribed as an initial and long-term therapy in Sjögren's. While hydroxychloroquine is an old drug that has been used successfully in rheumatic diseases for many years and is generally considered very safe and effective, a rare side effect of this drug can be retinal damage, so the most appropriate dose for each individual should be considered carefully along with regular monitoring by an ocular specialist.

Methotrexate (examples include Trexall®, Rheumatrex®)

This drug might or might not be prescribed at the same time as hydroxychloroquine.

The following DMARDs might be tried in any potential order and is dependent on physician preference and the individual patient:

Azathioprine (Imuran®)

Mycophenolate (examples include Cellcept®, Myfortic®)

Leflunomide (Arava®)

Cyclosporine (examples include Sandimmune®, Neoral®)

Dry Mouth Prescription Treatments

Evoxac® (cevimeline)

Salagen® (pilocarpine hydrochloride)

NeutraSal®

Dry Eye Prescription Treatments

Restasis® cyclosporine ophthalmic emulsion

Xiidra® lifitegrast ophthalmic solution

CEQUA™   Cyclosporine Ophthalmic Solution

TYRVAYA™ Varenicline Solution

Role of Inflammation: Explaining how inflammation exacerbates symptoms and affects overall health.

Inflammation is your body's response to an illness, injury or something that doesn't belong in your body (like germs or toxic chemicals). Inflammation is a normal and important process that allows your body to heal. Fever, for example, is how you know your body's inflammatory system is working correctly when you're ill. But inflammation can harm you if it occurs in healthy tissues or goes on for too long.

When an invader (like a virus) tries to enter your body, or you get injured, your immune system sends out its first responders. These are inflammatory cells and cytokines (substances that stimulate more inflammatory cells). These cells begin an inflammatory response to trap germs or toxins and start healing injured tissue. Inflammation can cause pain, swelling or discoloration. These are signs your body is healing itself. Normal inflammation should be mild, and pain shouldn't be extreme.

But inflammation can also affect parts of your body you can't see. Inflammatory responses that occur behind the scenes can help you heal, but other times, they can harm your health.

Types of Inflammation

There are two types of inflammation: acute and chronic.

Acute inflammation is the body's immediate response to an injury or infection. When the body is damaged, the immune system sends white blood cells to destroy any damaging substances, heal the tissues, and return the affected area to a state of balance. This rapid response causes familiar symptoms like redness, pain, warmth, and swelling. Acute inflammation usually resolves within a few hours to days.

Chronic inflammation can begin via the same process as acute inflammation but becomes persistent. It can happen in several ways. One possibility is that the threat remains because the body can't rid itself of the offending substance. Another scenario is that the immune system goes into "threat mode" when no actual threat exists. As a result, rather than healing tissues, the body breaks them down. Unhealthful lifestyle choices, such as smoking, a poor diet, excessive alcohol consumption, sedentary behavior, stress, and weight gain also can contribute to chronic inflammation.

Is inflammation helpful or harmful?

It turns out inflammation is both good and bad. On the one hand, acute inflammation helps the body to repair tissue damage and fight infections. Yet there is another side of inflammation that can be harmful rather than helpful to human health. A growing body of evidence suggests that low-grade, chronic inflammation contributes to some of the nation's leading killers, including cardiovascular disease, cancer, and type 2 diabetes as well as Alzheimer's disease, allergies and asthma, arthritis, anxiety and depression, and some skin conditions.

Where does inflammation occur?

Chronic inflammation can attack the entire body and, in the process, raise the risk for certain types of diseases and disorders in specific areas like the heart, brain, joints, and gastrointestinal tract.

Heart: Inflammation can raise the risk of heart attacks, and the link is believed to be related to cholesterol. Cholesterol can cause plaque build-up in the arteries, potentially blocking blood flow and leading to a heart attack. As cholesterol invades the wall of an artery, the immune system treats it like any other invader and releases inflammation-producing chemicals to help remove it. A fibrous cap is formed over the plaque. Inflammation inside the plaque can eventually eat away at the cap, and if it ruptures, the cholesterol, inflammatory cells, and chemicals in the plaque spill into the artery causing a blood clot to form which blocks blood flow.

Brain: Research has found that high amounts of inflammation in the body are associated with brain aging, increased cognitive decline, and "brain fog," which can impair thinking and cause memory lapses and confusion. Inflammation also may play a role in the production of an abnormal protein called tau, which is associated with Alzheimer's disease.

Joints: Chronic inflammation can lead to pain, swelling, stiffness, and joint damage, known as inflammatory arthritis. This can damage cartilage, bones, tendons (which attach muscle to bones), or ligaments (which hold joints together) and irritate nerves. Common types of inflammatory arthritis include rheumatoid arthritis, gout, and psoriatic arthritis.

Gastrointestinal tract: Inflammation is a driver of inflammatory bowel disease (IBD), a chronic inflammation of the gastrointestinal (GI) tract, including the stomach, gallbladder, and small and large intestines. Two types of IBD are ulcerative colitis, marked by continuous inflammation of the large intestine, and Crohn's disease, which causes inflammation anywhere in the GI tract. People with IBD can experience various symptoms, such as abdominal pain, diarrhea, blood in their stool, bloating, and weight loss.

Liver inflammation: Nonalcoholic fatty liver disease is fatty liver not caused by alcohol intake. There are two types: simple fatty liver and nonalcoholic steatohepatitis (NASH). Simple fatty liver doesn't cause inflammation. However, NASH is more severe and occurs when fattened cells become inflamed. This inflammation can damage liver cells, resulting in cirrhosis (permanent scarring of the liver), and increase the risk of liver cancer. Chronic liver inflammation can also be caused by a hepatitis C infection and lead to cirrhosis.

How do you reduce inflammation?

Although inflammation is vital to the body's defense and repair systems, chronic inflammation can cause more harm than good. That may make you wonder: what can I do about it? There are actually several ways to treat and reduce chronic inflammation. For example:

Follow a healthy, anti-inflammatory diet. Eating foods that have an anti-inflammatory effect may reduce inflammation and lower the risk of chronic illnesses associated with inflammation. Foods that reduce inflammation include:

Tomatoes

Olive oil

Green leafy vegetables, such as spinach, kale, and collards

Nuts like almonds and walnuts

Fatty fish like salmon, mackerel, tuna, and sardines

Whole grains such as quinoa, whole-grain bread, and oatmeal

Fruits such as strawberries, blueberries, and oranges

These foods contain high amounts of anti-inflammatory compounds and antioxidants like carotenoids, polyphenols, and omega-3 fatty acids.

An easy way to eat more anti-inflammatory foods is to follow an eating plan like the Mediterranean and MIND diets, which emphasize these foods. Following an anti-inflammatory diet also helps you avoid unhealthy foods that can cause inflammation, such as refined carbohydrates, such as white bread and pastries, processed foods, sugar-sweetened beverages, and red meat. High amounts of these foods also contribute to weight gain, another risk factor for inflammation.

Other ways you can reduce inflammation include:

Regular exercise: Moderate-intensity exercise can help prevent excess weight gain and manage cytokine levels. Cytokines are small proteins that play an essential role in normal immune responses, but large amounts can lead to inflammation.

Manage stress: Repeated bouts of stress can expose the body to high levels of cortisol (the stress hormone) and lead to chronic inflammation. Yoga, deep breathing, meditation, and other forms of relaxation can help calm your nervous system.

Medications: Anti-inflammatory medicines can help treat inflammatory conditions. Examples include corticosteroids and over-the-counter nonsteroidal anti-inflammatory drugs, such as Ibuprofen and naproxen. Speak with your doctor about whether medication is an option because they could cause side effects.

PART 2: PRINCIPLES OF AN ANTI-INFLAMMATORY DIET

An anti-inflammatory diet is designed to reduce chronic inflammation, a key factor in various health conditions such as Sjogren's syndrome. By focusing on specific nutrients and foods, this diet can play a crucial role in managing and alleviating inflammation-related symptoms.

Dietary Principles

To manage inflammation, it is essential to adopt dietary principles that support overall health.

A diet centered on whole, minimally processed foods is ideal.

This includes an ample variety of fruits and vegetables, which provide antioxidants and phytochemicals that help mitigate inflammation.

Whole grains are also a cornerstone of an anti-inflammatory diet as they are high in fiber, which aids in digestion and can help reduce inflammatory markers.

Consumption of proteins should be from lean sources, including fish rich in omega-3 fatty acids, like salmon and mackerel, which are known for their anti-inflammatory properties.

In addition to fish, other healthy protein sources such as legumes (beans, lentils) and nuts and seeds are encouraged.

Olive oil, a monounsaturated fat, is recommended as the primary fat source due to its potential to reduce inflammation.

Incorporating spices like turmeric, known for its curcumin content, can further assist in reducing inflammation.

This diet minimizes the intake of processed foods, sugary beverages, and refined carbohydrates, as these can exacerbate inflammation.

Foods to Include

Mediterranean Diet: This diet emphasizes consuming fruits, vegetables, whole grains, legumes, nuts, and seeds.

It is also rich in mono- and polyunsaturated fats, such as those found in olive oil, which are known to have anti-inflammatory properties. Here are the components that should be included liberally:

Omega-3 Fatty Acids: Found in fatty fish, flaxseeds, and walnuts, omega-3s help reduce inflammation.

Antioxidants: Fruits and vegetables, like berries and leafy greens, are packed with antioxidants which combat inflammation.

Recommended Foods:

Fruits and Vegetables: Focus on a variety, including leafy greens and berries for their anti-inflammatory benefits.

Whole Grains: Opt for grains like quinoa, brown rice, and oats, which are less likely to promote inflammation.

Healthy Fats: Include sources of healthy fats such as avocados, olive oil, and nuts.

Foods to Avoid

Processed Foods and Saturated Fats: These foods can exacerbate inflammation and should be limited in an anti-inflammatory diet. This includes:

Processed Food: Anything heavily processed or with added preservatives should be avoided.

Saturated Fat: Foods high in saturated fat like butter and fatty cuts of meat can increase inflammation.

Salt: Excessive salt intake can worsen inflammation and strain on blood vessels.

Refined Sugars and Simple Carbohydrates: Consumption of these can lead to spikes in blood sugar and insulin levels, which may trigger an inflammatory response.

Specific Avoidances:

Sugar: Minimize intake of sugars that can prompt an inflammatory process.

Cookies and Sweets: These often contain both refined sugars and saturated fats, which are best avoided in an anti-inflammatory diet.

PART 3: KEY NUTRIENTS FOR MANAGING SJÖGREN'S SYNDROME

When adhering to an anti-inflammatory diet, focus on the following key nutrients and foods:

Omega-3 Fatty Acids

Omega-3 fatty acids are a type of polyunsaturated fat — also referred to as "healthy fats" — praised for their potential protective roles in several chronic diseases, such as heart disease and dementia.

They are one of the key building blocks for cell membranes and remain a subject of interest in the scientific community.

The family of omega-3 fatty acids includes:

Alpha-linolenic acid (ALA)

Stearidonic acid (SDA)

Eicosapentaenoic acid (EPA)

Docosapentaenoic acid (DPA)

Docosahexaenoic acid (DHA)

DHA and EPA are the primary polyunsaturated fats in brain cell membranes and have been popularized and successfully marketed as dietary supplements.

Omega-3 fatty acids are essential, meaning the human body is incapable of creating them on its own — the fatty acids or their precursors must be obtained from the diet.

For instance, ALA from plant seeds can be converted in the body to all the other types of omega-3 fats: EPA, SDA, DHA, DPA.

Studies have shown that increasing the levels of omega-3s in our cell membranes may protect against or help to reduce the symptoms of certain diseases. For example, scientists have discovered that increasing the Omega-3 Index can decrease the risk of death in patients with heart disease and can decrease swollen joints in patients with rheumatoid arthritis. One thing that these ailments have in common is inflammation, which can be reduced by omega-3s.

In many cases, inflammation is a very good thing. It is the process that occurs when the immune system fights back against an infection. Have you ever gotten a splinter, and noticed that the area is swollen, redder than the rest of your skin, and maybe a bit painful? This is inflammation! Your immune system is working hard to fight off any bacteria that may have entered your body when you got the splinter. Normally, once your immune system has eliminated the threat of an infection, the area will heal and return to normal. Unfortunately, sometimes this process goes haywire and inflammation can continue when it is not necessary. This is referred to as chronic inflammation, and it can have many negative effects, including permanent damage to the tissue. Medical concerns including heart disease, arthritis, and even some cancers are associated with chronic inflammation, which is why it is so important to keep inflammation from getting out of control.

Scientists have shown that a high Omega-3 Index can help protect against chronic or uncontrolled inflammation. Specifically, maintaining a proper balance of omega-3s and omega-6s in the diet is critical for maintaining healthy omega-3 levels in the cell membranes. It is important to remember that nutrition is all about balance: we don't want to consume only omega-3s, but instead we should try to eat a healthy proportion of both omega-3s and omega-6s. Scientists recommend that we eat only about 2 times more omega-6s than omega-3s, but it is estimated that most Americans consume more than 20 times more omega-6s than omega-3s. This imbalance in dietary fatty acids may contribute to the chronic inflammatory diseases prevalent in individuals consuming a Western-style diet.

How do omega-3s help reduce inflammation?

This is a question that scientists are still trying to understand, but there are a few discoveries that could explain this. First, having more omega-3s in their cell membranes allows cells to make more omega-3-derived metabolites, many of which can turn off the inflammatory response and turn on a healing response that helps the tissue or cell repair any damage caused by inflammation. Another way omega-3s reduce inflammation could be through changes in types and amounts of microorganisms that live in the gut, called the gut microbiota. It is well known that what we choose to eat influences the microorganisms that live in the gut and that these organisms can influence our health. Scientists have found that consuming omega-3 fatty acids changes the types of microbes in the gut, but it is not yet known exactly how these changes to the microbiota influence inflammation. These are just two of many potential ways that omega-3s can protect against inflammation.

Omega-3 fats: What they can do for health

Decades of research on the health impacts of omega-3 fatty acids have provided controversial findings. Here are some evidence-backed benefits of consuming omega-3 fatty acids.

Anti-inflammatory properties

Chronic inflammation — also called low-grade inflammation — is linked to the development of obesity, heart disease, and cancers.

Omega-3 fatty acids have been shown to exert anti-inflammatory effects in the human body and may aid in lowering markers of inflammation, such as C-reactive protein and interleukin-6.

In fact, omega-3 fatty acids are regarded as one of the most potent lipids capable of reducing oxidative stress and inflammation. It also potentially guards against the development of chronic diseases.

Lower cholesterol

In a 6-week study, daily supplementation with at least 1.2 g of DHA significantly reduced triglyceride levels and increased "good" cholesterol, or high-density lipoprotein.

In addition, omega-3 fatty acids lowered the "bad" cholesterol, low-density lipoproteins (LDL), when dietary saturated fats were replaced with polyunsaturated and monounsaturated fatty acids found in plants foods such as nuts and avocados.

Elevated triglycerides and LDL cholesterol are linked to an increased risk for metabolic syndrome and heart disease.

However, a recent evidence-based practice summary has shown no impact on a range of cardiovascular disease (CVD) outcomes from the use of omega-3 fatty acid supplements in patients with established CVD or raised risk factors for CVD.

Lower blood pressure

On the other hand, omega-3 fatty acids have been shown to improve vascular health — the health of the blood vessels — by increasing the bioavailability of nitric oxide.

In a phase 2 scientific study, nitric oxide induced dilation (relaxation) of the blood vessels and led to a significant reduction in blood pressure.

May reduce the risk of heart disease

By reducing markers associated with an increased risk of developing heart disease — high triglycerides, cholesterol, and blood pressure — omega-3 fatty acids may reduce the risk of heart disease, according to a review analyzing existing studies.

The same review concluded that high-dose daily supplementation with 4 g of purified EPA in people with elevated triglycerides levels led to a 25% reduction in cardiovascular events.

In their 2018 review, Prof. Fereidoon Shahidi, professor of biochemistry at Memorial University, Canada, and Prof. Priyatharini Ambigaipalan, currently at the School of Science and Engineering Technology at Durham College, also in Canada, identified evidence of health benefits from omega-3 in noncardiovascular health conditions.

Improve tolerance to cancer treatment

Omega-3 fatty acids may improve the efficacy and tolerance of chemotherapy and is a potential supportive treatment to people undergoing cancer treatment.

More specifically, daily supplementation with EPA and DHA helped patients with head and neck cancers and breast cancer to maintain body weight and reduce cancer-related muscle loss.

Improves depression

A 2019 review study of over 2,000 participants showed a beneficial impact of EPA omega-3 fatty acids on depression, with DHA showing little benefits.

This finding is supported by other studies by experts, indicating that fish oil supplementation helps protect against major depressive disorder in people between the ages of 15 and 25 years.

Furthermore, moderate intakes of fatty fish and seafood were associated with fewer occurrences of depression.

Foods with Omega-3 Fatty Acids

When possible, try to get your omega-3 fatty acids from foods rather than supplements.

Fish high in omega-3s

Aim to eat nonfried, oily fish high in DHA and EPA at least two times a week. Here are several:

Anchovies

Bluefish

Flounder

Freshwater trout

Herring

Salmon

Sardines

Sturgeon

Tuna

While eating more fatty fish is good, some are likely to have higher levels of mercury, polychlorinated biphenyls, or other toxins. These include bigeye tuna, mackerel, wild swordfish, tilefish, and shark.

Vegan sources of omega-3s

Beans

Canola oil

Chia seeds

Edamame

Flaxseed and flaxseed oil

Soybean oil

Walnuts

Bear in mind that oils and nuts can be high in calories, so eat them in moderation.

Antioxidants: Role in combating oxidative stress and supporting immune function.

Antioxidants can prevent or slow cell damage caused by free radicals, which are unstable molecules that the body produces as a reaction to environmental and other pressures.

Free radicals can increase the risk of inflammation and various health issues. They are sometimes called "free-radical scavengers."

The sources of antioxidants can be natural or artificial. Certain plant-based foods are thought to be rich in antioxidants. Plant-based antioxidants are a kind of phytonutrient, or plant-based nutrient.

The body also produces some antioxidants, known as endogenous antioxidants. Antioxidants that come from outside the body are called exogenous.

Free radicals are waste substances produced by cells as the body processes food and reacts to the environment. If the body cannot process and remove free radicals efficiently, oxidative stress can result. This can harm cells and body function. Free radicals are also known as reactive oxygen species (ROS).

Factors that increase the production of free radicals in the body can be internal, such as inflammation, or external, for example, pollution, UV exposure, and cigarette smoke.

Oxidative stress has been linked to heart disease, cancer, arthritis, stroke, respiratory diseases, immune deficiency, emphysema, Parkinson's disease, and other inflammatory or ischemic conditions.

Antioxidants are said to help neutralize free radicals in our bodies, and this is thought to boost overall health.

Benefits

Antioxidants can protect against the cell damage that free radicals cause, known as oxidative stress.

Activities and processes that can lead to oxidative stress include:

Mitochondrial activity

Excessive exercise

Tissue trauma, due to inflammation and injury

Ischemia and reperfusion damage

Consumption of certain foods, especially refined and processed foods, trans fats, artificial sweeteners, and certain dyes and additives

Smoking

Environmental pollution

Radiation

Exposure to chemicals, such as pesticides and drugs, including chemotherapy

Industrial solvents

Ozone

Such activities and exposures can result in cell damage.

This, in turn, may lead to:

An excessive release of free iron or copper ions

An activation of phagocytes, a type of white blood cell with a role in fighting infection

An increase in enzymes that generate free radicals

A disruption of electron transport chains

All these can result in oxidative stress.

The damage caused by oxidative stress has been linked to cancer, atherosclerosis, and vision loss. It is thought that the free radicals cause changes in the cells that lead to these and possibly other conditions.

An intake of antioxidants is believed to reduce these risks.

According to one study: "Antioxidants act as radical scavenger, hydrogen donor, electron donor, peroxide decomposer, singlet oxygen quencher, enzyme inhibitor, synergist, and metal-chelating agents."

Other research has indicated that antioxidant supplements may help reduce vision loss due to age-related macular degeneration in older people.

Overall, however, there is a lack of evidence that a higher intake of specific antioxidants can reduce the risk of disease. In most cases, results have tended to show no benefit, or a detrimental effect, or they have been conflicting.

Types

There are thought to be hundreds and possibly thousands of substances that can act as antioxidants. Each has its own role and can interact with others to help the body work effectively.

"Antioxidant" is not really the name of a substance, but rather it describes what a range of substances can do.

Examples of antioxidants that come from outside the body include:

Vitamin A

Vitamin C

Vitamin E

Beta-Carotene

Lycopene

Lutein

Selenium

Manganese

Zeaxanthin

Flavonoids, flavones, catechins, polyphenols, and phytoestrogens are all types of antioxidants and phytonutrients, and they are all found in plant-based foods.

Each antioxidant serves a different function and is not interchangeable with another. This is why it is important to have a varied diet.

Food sources

The best sources of antioxidants are plant-based foods, especially fruits and vegetables.

Foods that are particularly high in antioxidants are often referred to as a "superfood" or "functional food."

To obtain some specific antioxidants, try to include the following in your diet:

Vitamin A: Dairy produce, eggs, and liver

Vitamin C: Most fruits and vegetables, especially berries, oranges, and bell peppers

Vitamin E: Nuts and seeds, sunflower and other vegetable oils, and green, leafy vegetables

Beta-carotene: Brightly colored fruits and vegetables, such as carrots, peas, spinach, and mangoes

Lycopene: Pink and red fruits and vegetables, including tomatoes and watermelon

Lutein: Green, leafy vegetables, corn, papaya, and oranges

Selenium: Rice, corn, wheat, and other whole grains, as well as nuts, eggs, cheese, and legumes

Other foods that are believed to be good sources of antioxidants include:

Eggplants

Legumes such as black beans or kidney beans

Green and black teas

Red grapes

Dark chocolate

Pomegranates

Goji berries.

Foods with rich, vibrant colors often contain the most antioxidants.

The following foods are good sources of antioxidants.

Blueberries

Apples

Broccoli

Spinach

Lentils

Vitamin D: Importance in autoimmune conditions and ways to ensure adequate intake.

Vitamin D is a fat-soluble vitamin in a family of compounds that includes vitamins D1, D2, and D3.

Your body produces vitamin D naturally when it's directly exposed to sunlight. You can also get vitamin D from certain foods and supplements to ensure adequate levels of the vitamin in your blood.

Vitamin D has several important functions. Perhaps the most vital are regulating the absorption of calcium and phosphorus and facilitating healthy immune system function.

Getting enough vitamin D is important for the typical growth and development of bones and teeth and for improving resistance to certain diseases.

In respect to autoimmune diseases, although the cause of most autoimmune disease is largely unknown, the leading theory is that the regulation of the body's immune system goes awry. The immune system normally defends the body from invaders such as infections, and helps repair damaged tissues. When an autoimmune condition develops, the immune system attacks its host. For example, with rheumatoid arthritis, immune cells attack joints, lungs, and other parts of the body.

Research has shown that vitamin D can interact with immune cells, affect genes that regulate inflammation, and alter the response of the immune system.

Here is more information about the benefits of vitamin D, its downsides, how much you need, and foods with vitamin D.

1. **Vitamin D may fight disease**

In addition to its primary benefits, research suggests that vitamin D may also play a role in:

Reducing the risk of multiple sclerosis (MS): A 2017 review of population-based studies found that low levels of vitamin D are linked with an increased risk of MS.

Decreasing the chance of heart disease: Low vitamin D levels have been linked to increased risk of heart diseases such as hypertension, heart failure, and stroke. However, it's unclear whether vitamin D deficiency contributes to heart disease or indicates poor health when you have a chronic condition.

Reducing the likelihood of severe illnesses: Although studies are mixed, vitamin D may make severe flu and COVID-19 infections less likely. A recent review found that low vitamin D levels contribute to acute respiratory distress syndrome.

Supporting immune health: People who do not have adequate vitamin D levels might be at increased risk of infections and autoimmune diseases, such as rheumatoid arthritis, type 1 diabetes, and inflammatory bowel disease.

2. May regulate mood and reduce depression

Research has shown that vitamin D might play an important role in regulating mood and decreasing the risk of depression.

A review of 7,534 people found that those experiencing negative emotions who received vitamin D supplements noticed an improvement in symptoms. Vitamin D supplementation may help people with depression who also have a vitamin D deficiency.

Another study identified low vitamin D levels as a risk factor for more severe fibromyalgia symptoms, anxiety, and depression.

3. May support weight loss

People with higher body weights have a greater chance of low vitamin D levels, and some studies suggest there may be a link between vitamin D and obesity, though more research is needed to verify this.

In an older study, people taking daily calcium and vitamin D supplements lost more weight than subjects taking a placebo supplement. The researchers suggest that the extra calcium and vitamin D may have had an appetite-suppressing effect.

Current research doesn't support the idea that vitamin D causes weight loss, but there appears to be a relationship between vitamin D and weight.

Probiotics: Gut health and its connection to inflammation and autoimmune responses.

The bacteria in your body are said to outnumber your body's cells at a 10-to-1 ratio. However, a recent study says that the ratio is closer to 1-to-1.

According to these estimates, you have 39–300 trillion bacteria living inside you. Whichever estimate is most accurate, it's certainly a large number.

Much of these bacteria reside in your gut, and the majority are quite harmless. Some are helpful, and a small number can cause disease.

Having the right gut bacteria has been linked to numerous health benefits, including the following:

Weight loss

Improved digestion

Enhanced immune function

Healthier skin

Reduced risk of some diseases

Probiotics, which are a certain type of friendly bacteria, provide health benefits when eaten.

They're often taken as supplements that are supposed to help colonize your gut with good microorganisms.

What are probiotics?

Probiotics are living microorganisms that, when ingested, provide a health benefit.

However, the scientific community often disagrees on what the benefits are, as well as which strains of bacteria are responsible.

Probiotics are usually bacteria, but certain types of yeasts can also function as probiotics. There are also other microorganisms in the gut that are being studied, including viruses, fungi, archaea, and helminths.

You can get probiotics from supplements, as well as from foods prepared by bacterial fermentation.

Probiotic foods include yogurt, kefir, sauerkraut, tempeh, and kimchi. Probiotics should not be confused with prebiotics, which are carbs — often dietary fibers — that help feed the friendly bacteria already in your gut.

Products that contain both prebiotics and probiotics are referred to as synbiotics. Synbiotic products usually combine friendly bacteria along with some food for the bacteria to eat (the prebiotics), all in one supplement.

The most common probiotic bacteria are Lactobacillus and Bifidobacteria. Other common kinds are Saccharomyces, Streptococcus, Enterococcus, Escherichia, and Bacillus.

Each genus comprises different species, and each species has many strains. On labels, you'll see probiotics identified by their specific strain (which includes the genus), the species, subspecies if there is one, and a letter-number strain code.

Different probiotics have been found to address different health conditions. Therefore, choosing the right type — or types — of probiotics is essential.

Some supplements, known as broad-spectrum probiotics or multi-probiotics, combine different species in the same product.

Although the evidence is promising, more research is needed on the health benefits of probiotics. Some researchers warn about possible negative effects from the "dark side" of probiotics and call for caution and strict regulation.

Importance of microorganisms for your gut

The complex community of microorganisms in your gut is called the gut flora, gut microbiota, or gut microbiome.

The gut microbiota includes bacteria, viruses, fungi, archaea, and helminths — with bacteria comprising the vast majority. Your gut is home to a complex eco-system of 300–500 bacterial species.

Most of the gut flora is found in your colon, or large intestine, which is the last part of your digestive tract.

Surprisingly, the metabolic activities of your gut flora resemble those of an organ. For this reason, some scientists refer to the gut flora as the "forgotten organ".

Your gut flora performs many important health functions. It manufactures vitamins, including vitamin K and some of the B vitamins.

It also turns fibers into short-chain fats like butyrate, propionate, and acetate, which feed your gut wall and perform many metabolic functions.

These fats also stimulate your immune system and strengthen your gut wall. This can help prevent unwanted substances from entering your body and provoking an immune response.

Your gut flora is highly sensitive to your diet, and studies show that an unbalanced gut flora is linked to numerous diseases.

These diseases are thought to include obesity, type 2 diabetes, metabolic syndrome, heart disease, colorectal cancer, Alzheimer's, and depression.

Probiotics and prebiotic fibers can help correct this balance, ensuring that your "forgotten organ" is functioning optimally.

Impact on digestive health

Probiotics are widely researched for their effects on digestive health.

Evidence suggests that probiotic supplements can help cure antibiotic-associated diarrhea.

When people take antibiotics, especially for long periods of time, they often experience diarrhea — even long after the infection has been eradicated.

This is because the antibiotics kill many of the natural bacteria in your gut, which shifts the gut balance and allows harmful bacteria to thrive.

Probiotics may also help combat irritable bowel syndrome (IBS), a common digestive disorder, reducing gas, bloating, constipation, diarrhea, and other symptoms.

Impact on weight loss

Some research indicates that people with obesity have different gut bacteria than those who are lean.

Research shows a connection between gut microbes and obesity in both infants and adults. It also shows that microbial changes in the gut are a factor in developing obesity as an adult.

Therefore, many scientists believe that your gut bacteria are important in determining body weight.

While more research is needed, some probiotic strains appear to aid weight loss.

Nevertheless, researchers advise caution in rushing to this conclusion, noting that there are still many unknowns.

These unknowns include:

The specific strains of probiotics to be used

The dosage and duration of treatment

The long-term effects of treatment

The interaction of age, gender, health conditions, and lifestyle

In one study, 210 people with central obesity, which is characterized by excess belly fat, took the probiotic Lactobacillus gasseri daily. Participants lost an average of approximately 8.5 % of their belly fat over 12 weeks.

When participants stopped taking the probiotic, they gained the belly fat back within 4 weeks.

Evidence also suggests that Lactobacillus rhamnosus and Bifidobacterium lactis can aid weight loss and help prevent obesity — though more research is needed.

Other health benefits

There are many other benefits of probiotics. They may help with the following conditions:

Inflammation: Probiotics reduce systemic inflammation, a leading driver of many diseases.

Depression and anxiety: The probiotic strains Lactobacillus helveticus and Bifidobacterium longum have been shown to reduce symptoms of anxiety and depression in people with clinical depression.

Blood cholesterol: Several probiotics have been shown to lower total and LDL (bad) cholesterol levels, although the research remains controversial.

Blood pressure: Probiotics may also cause modest reductions in blood pressure.

Immune function: Several probiotic strains may enhance immune function, possibly leading to a reduced risk of infections, including those that cause the common cold.

Skin health: There's some evidence that probiotics can be useful for acne, rosacea, and eczema, as well as other skin disorders.

Anti-aging: Though research is extremely limited, there's evidence that probiotics have the potential to extend lifespan by increasing the ability of cells to replicate themselves.

This is only a small slice of probiotics' benefits, as ongoing studies indicate a wide breadth of potential health effects.

PART 4: TASTY, YUMMY RECIPES FOR AN ANTI-INFLAMMATORY SJÖGREN DIET

RECIPES FOR BREAKFAST ON THE ANTI-INFLAMMATORY SJÖGREN DIET

Baked Eggs with Roasted Vegetables

Ingredients

3 cups small broccoli florets (about 1 inch in size)

12 ounces yellow potatoes, such as Yukon Gold, cut into 1/2- to 3/4-inch pieces (about 2 cups)

1 large sweet potato, cut into 1/2- to 3/4-inch pieces (about 1 cup)

1 small red onion, cut into thin slices

2 tablespoons olive oil

6 eggs

2 ounces Manchego cheese, shredded (1/2 cup)

½ teaspoon cracked black pepper

Directions

1. Preheat oven to 425 degrees Fahrenheit. Coat a 2-quart rectangular baking dish with nonstick cooking spray. In a large bowl combine broccoli, yellow potatoes, sweet potato, onion, olive oil and 1/4 teaspoon salt, tossing to coat vegetables.
2. Spread vegetable mixture evenly in the prepared pan. Roast for 10 minutes. Stir vegetables; roast

about 5 minutes more or until vegetables are tender and starting to brown. Remove from oven. Spread vegetables evenly in baking dish; cool. Cover and chill in the refrigerator for 8 to 24 hours.

3. Let chilled vegetables stand at room temperature for 30 minutes. Meanwhile, preheat oven to 375 degrees Fahrenheit.

4. Bake vegetables, uncovered, for 5 minutes. Remove from oven; make six wells in the layer of vegetables. Break an egg into each well. Bake for 5 minutes more. Sprinkle with cheese. Bake for 5 to 10 minutes more or until eggs whites are set and yolks are starting to thicken. Sprinkle with pepper.

Pineapple Green Smoothie

Ingredients

½ cup unsweetened almond milk

⅓ cup nonfat plain Greek yogurt

1 cup baby spinach

1 cup frozen banana slices (about 1 medium banana)

½ cup frozen pineapple chunks

1 tablespoon chia seeds

1-2 teaspoons pure maple syrup or honey (optional)

Directions

Add almond milk and yogurt to a blender, then add spinach, banana, pineapple, chia seeds and sweetener (if using); blend until smooth.

Apple-Cinnamon Quinoa Bowl

Ingredients

¾ cup low-fat milk

⅔ cup diced apple, divided

¼ cup quinoa

¼ teaspoon ground cinnamon

⅛ teaspoon salt

4 teaspoons sliced almonds

½ teaspoon honey

Directions

1. Combine milk, 1/3 cup apple, quinoa, cinnamon and salt in a small saucepan. Bring to a boil.

Cover and simmer on very low heat until the liquid is absorbed, about 12 minutes.

2. Let stand 5 minutes. Top with the remaining 1/3 cup apple, almonds and honey.

Banana Oatmeal

Ingredients

4 large ripe bananas, divided

3 cups low-fat milk

2 cups old-fashioned rolled oats (see Tip)

3 tablespoons pure maple syrup

1 teaspoon vanilla extract

¾ teaspoon ground cinnamon, plus more for sprinkling

¼ teaspoon ground ginger

⅛ teaspoon salt

Directions

Peel and slice 1 banana; reserve for serving. Using a fork, mash the remaining 3 bananas in a large saucepan. Add milk and bring the mixture to a simmer over medium-high heat, scraping the bottom of the pan often with a wooden spoon. Stir in oats, maple syrup, vanilla, cinnamon, ginger and salt. Reduce heat to medium-low. Cook, scraping the bottom of the pan often with the spoon, until the mixture is thick and creamy, about 5 minutes. Divide the oatmeal evenly among 4 bowls; top evenly with the reserved banana slices. Sprinkle with cinnamon, if desired, and serve immediately.

Summer Skillet Vegetable & Egg Scramble

Ingredients

2 tablespoons olive oil

12 ounces baby potatoes, thinly sliced

4 cups thinly sliced vegetables, such as mushrooms, bell peppers, and/or zucchini (14 oz.)

3 scallions, thinly sliced, green and white parts separated

1 teaspoon minced fresh herbs, such as rosemary or thyme

6 large eggs (or 4 large eggs plus 4 egg whites), lightly beaten

2 cups packed leafy greens, such as baby spinach or baby kale (2 oz.)

½ teaspoon salt

Directions

1. Heat oil in a large cast-iron or nonstick skillet over medium heat. Add potatoes; cover and cook, stirring several times, until they begin to soften, about 8 minutes.

2. Add sliced vegetables and scallion whites; cook uncovered, stirring occasionally, until the vegetables are tender and lightly browned, 8 to 10 minutes. Stir in herbs. Move the vegetable mixture to the perimeter of the pan.

3. Reduce heat to medium-low. Add eggs and scallion greens to the center of the pan. Cook, stirring, until the eggs are softly scrambled, about 2 minutes.

4. Stir leafy greens into the eggs. Remove from heat and stir to combine well. Stir in salt.

Berry Chia Pudding

Ingredients

1 ¾ cups blackberries, raspberries and/or diced mango (fresh or frozen), divided

1 cup unsweetened almond milk or milk of choice

¼ cup chia seeds

1 tablespoon pure maple syrup

¾ teaspoon vanilla extract

½ cup whole-milk plain Greek yogurt

¼ cup granola

Directions

1. Puree 1 1/4 cups fruit and milk in a blender or food processor until smooth. Scrape into a

medium bowl; mix in chia, syrup and vanilla. Cover and refrigerate for at least 8 hours and up to 3 days.

2. Divide the pudding between 2 bowls, layering each serving with 1/4 cup of the remaining fruit, 1/4 cup yogurt and 2 tablespoons granola.

Sweet Potato, Broccoli & Wild Rice Hash

Ingredients

2 tablespoons extra-virgin olive oil plus 1 teaspoon, divided

1 pound sweet potato (1 large), peeled and cut into 1/2-inch pieces (3 1/2 cups)

½ teaspoon salt, divided

2 cups small broccoli florets

3 small spring onions or scallions, sliced, whites and greens separated, divided

1 clove garlic, minced

1 cup cooked wild rice or wild rice blend (see Tip)

2 tablespoons chopped flat-leaf parsley

2 tablespoons finely chopped fresh tarragon

4 large eggs

Directions

1. Heat 1 tablespoon oil in a large cast-iron or nonstick skillet over medium heat. Add sweet potatoes and season with 1/4 teaspoon salt. Cook, stirring often, until lightly browned and softened, 8 to 10 minutes. Add broccoli and 1 tablespoon oil; cook, stirring occasionally, until softened, 3 to 5 minutes. Add spring onion (or scallion) whites and garlic; cook, stirring, for 1 minute. Stir in rice, spring onion (or scallion) greens, parsley and tarragon and remove from heat. Transfer to a plate and cover to keep warm.

2. Heat the remaining 1 teaspoon oil in the pan over medium heat. Crack eggs into the pan and season with the remaining 1/4 teaspoon salt.

Cook to desired doneness, 1 1/2 to 2 minutes for a runny yolk and 3 1/2 to 4 minutes for a firmer yolk. Serve the eggs on top of the hash.

Spinach-Avocado Smoothie

Ingredients

1 cup nonfat plain yogurt

1 cup fresh spinach

1 frozen banana

¼ avocado

2 tablespoons water

1 teaspoon honey

Directions

Combine yogurt, spinach, banana, avocado, water and honey in a blender. Puree until smooth

Overnight Matcha Oats with Berries

Ingredients

⅔ cup nonfat milk

⅔ cup old-fashioned oats (see Tip)

1 teaspoon matcha powder

1 tablespoon chia seeds

2 teaspoons pure maple syrup

⅛ teaspoon salt

¼ cup blueberries

¼ cup raspberries

1 tablespoon sliced almonds

Directions

Combine milk, oats, matcha powder, chia seeds, maple syrup and salt in a pint jar and stir. Top with blueberries, raspberries and almonds. Cover and refrigerate overnight.

Sriracha, Egg & Avocado Overnight Oats

Ingredients

½ cup rolled oats (see Tip)

¾ cup water

1 tablespoon onion

¼ avocado, sliced

2 cherry tomatoes, chopped

1 large egg, fried

1 teaspoon Sriracha

Directions

1. Combine oats and water in a small bowl or jar. Cover and refrigerate overnight.

2. Stir in onion and microwave in 30-second intervals, stirring occasionally, until heated through. Arrange in a bowl with avocado and tomatoes. Top with the egg and Sriracha.

English Muffin Pizza with Tomato & Olives

Ingredients

1 whole-wheat English muffin, split and toasted

1 medium tomato, sliced

1 tablespoon sliced green olives

2 tablespoons shredded mozzarella cheese

⅛ teaspoon dried oregano

Directions

1. Preheat broiler to high.
2. Top each English muffin half with half of the tomato slices, olives, cheese and oregano. Broil until the cheese is melted, about 2 minutes.

Overnight Quinoa Pudding

Ingredients

1 cup cooked and cooled quinoa

¾ cup plain kefir

1 tablespoon chia seeds, plus more for serving

2 teaspoons pure maple syrup

¼ teaspoon vanilla extract

Dash of ground cinnamon

1 cup Fresh berries for serving

Directions

Combine quinoa, kefir, chia seeds, maple syrup, vanilla and cinnamon in a bowl or jar. Refrigerate overnight. To serve, top with berries and more chia, if desired.

Anti-Inflammatory Cherry-Spinach Smoothie

Ingredients

1 cup plain low-fat kefir

1 cup frozen cherries

½ cup baby spinach leaves

¼ cup mashed ripe avocado

1 tablespoon salted almond butter

1 (1/2 inch) piece peeled ginger

1 teaspoon chia seeds, plus more for garnish

Directions

Place kefir in a blender. Add cherries, spinach, avocado, almond butter, ginger and chia seeds; puree until smooth. Pour into a glass; garnish with more chia seeds, if desired.

Good Green Tea Smoothie

Ingredients

3 cups frozen white grapes

2 packed cups baby spinach

1 1/2 cups strong brewed green tea (see Tip), cooled

1 medium ripe avocado

2 teaspoons honey

Directions

Combine grapes, spinach, green tea, avocado and honey in a blender; blend until smooth. Serve immediately.

Acai Bowl

Ingredients

1 banana

½ cup frozen mixed berries

1 (3.5-ounce) package frozen unsweetened acai puree

¼ cup fat-free plain strained yogurt, such as Greek-style

¼ cup coconut water

1 tablespoon almond butter

⅛ teaspoon ground cinnamon

2 tablespoons dried goji berries

2 tablespoons sliced almonds, toasted (see Tip)

1 teaspoon chia seeds

1 teaspoon hemp seeds

Directions

1. Cut banana in half crosswise; peel 1 half (set aside the remaining unpeeled half). Place the peeled banana half on a freezer-safe plate lined with parchment paper; freeze until solid, about 2 hours.

2. Place the frozen banana, berries, acai puree, yogurt, coconut water, almond butter and cinnamon in a blender. Blend until smooth, 30 to 45 seconds, stopping to scrape down sides of blender as needed. Peel and slice the reserved banana half.

3. Pour the smoothie into a bowl; top with the banana slices, goji berries, almonds, chia seeds and hemp seeds. Serve immediately.

RECIPES FOR LUNCH ON THE ANTI-INFLAMMATORY SJÖGREN DIET

Black Bean Fajita Skillet

Ingredients

1 tablespoon olive oil

1 (12-ounce) package sliced fajita vegetables (bell peppers and onions)

1 (15-ounce) can no-salt-added black beans, rinsed

½ teaspoon salt-free Southwest-style seasoning blend

¼ teaspoon salt

¼ cup coarsely shredded Cheddar cheese (1 ounce; optional)

Directions

1. Heat oil in a large skillet over medium heat. Add fajita vegetables and sauté until tender, about 10 minutes.
2. Stir in black beans, seasoning and salt; cook, stirring, until heated through, about 1 minute.
3. Divide the vegetables and beans between two bowls and top each with 2 tablespoons cheese, if using.

Fiber-Packed Spicy White Bean & Spinach Salad

Ingredients

2 (15-ounce) cans no-salt-added cannellini beans, rinsed

⅓ cup whole-milk plain yogurt

¾ teaspoon ras el hanout

½ teaspoon refrigerated garlic paste

½ teaspoon salt

½ teaspoon honey

2 tablespoons extra-virgin olive oil

1 tablespoon red-wine vinegar

1 tablespoon harissa paste

1 (5 ounce) package baby spinach

1 cup julienned carrots

¼ cup unsalted roasted almonds, chopped

3 tablespoons golden raisins

Directions

Combine beans, yogurt, ras el hanout, garlic paste, salt and honey in a medium bowl; stir to incorporate, coarsely mashing beans, if desired. Whisk oil, vinegar and harissa together in a large bowl. Add spinach, carrots, almonds and raisins; toss to coat. Serve the spinach mixture with the bean salad.

Cabbage, Tofu & Edamame Salad

Ingredients

4 cups mesclun

½ cup shredded red cabbage

3 ounces baked tofu cubes

½ cup grated carrots

½ cup edamame

¼ cup mandarin oranges

1 tablespoon golden raisins

½ cup bamboo shoots

2 tablespoons chow mein noodles

2 tablespoons bottled reduced-sugar Asian sesame vinaigrette

Directions

Mix mesclun, cabbage, tofu, carrots, edamame, oranges, raisins, bamboo shoots, and chow mein noodles in a medium bowl. Drizzle with vinaigrette.

Berry-Kefir Smoothie

Ingredients

1 ½ cups frozen mixed berries

1 cup plain kefir

½ medium banana

2 teaspoons almond butter

½ teaspoon vanilla extract

Directions

Combine berries, kefir, banana, almond butter and vanilla in a blender. Blend until smooth.

Spicy Ramen Noodle Cup Soup Packs 16g Protein

Ingredients

1 ½ tablespoons reduced-sodium vegetable bouillon paste

1 ½ teaspoons white miso

1 ½ teaspoons chile-garlic sauce

1 ½ teaspoons grated ginger

¾ cup shredded carrot

¾ cup sliced shiitake mushrooms

1 ½ cups chopped baby spinach

3 hard-boiled eggs, halved

1 ½ cups cooked ramen noodles

3 tablespoons sliced scallions

¾ teaspoon sesame seeds

3 cups very hot water, divided

Directions

1. Place 1/2 tablespoon bouillon paste, 1/2 teaspoon miso, 1/2 teaspoon chili-garlic sauce and 1/2

teaspoon ginger in each of 3 pint-and-a-half size canning jars. Layer 1/4 cup carrot, 1/4 cup mushrooms, 1/2 cup spinach, 2 egg halves and 1/2 cup noodles in each jar. Top each with 1 tablespoon scallions and 1/4 teaspoon sesame seeds. Close the jars. Refrigerate for up to 3 days.

2. To make one jar of noodles, add 1 cup of very hot water to one jar. Close the jar and shake to combine. Microwave uncovered on high in 1-minute increments until steaming hot, 2 to 3 minutes. Let stand 5 minutes. Stir before eating.

Cranberry-Walnut Chickpea Salad

Ingredients

¼ cup low-fat plain strained yogurt, such as Greek-style

1 tablespoon minced onion

2 teaspoons lemon juice

¼ teaspoon salt

1 (15 ounce) can no-salt-added chickpeas, rinsed

¼ cup diced celery

¼ cup dried cranberries

¼ cup chopped walnuts, toasted (see Tip)

Directions

Mix yogurt, onion, lemon juice and salt in a medium bowl. Add chickpeas, celery, cranberries and walnuts; toss to coat.

Butternut Squash Soup with Avocado & Chickpeas

Ingredients

1 15-ounce can Amy's Light-in-Sodium Butternut Squash Soup

¾ cup canned chickpeas, rinsed

1 tablespoon lime juice

1 teaspoon curry powder

Pinch of salt

2 tablespoons diced avocado

1 tablespoon nonfat plain Greek yogurt

Directions

Heat soup in a small saucepan with chickpeas, lime juice, curry powder and salt. To serve, top with avocado and yogurt.

Veggie Sandwich

Ingredients

2 slices sprouted-grain bread, toasted if desired

¼ avocado, mashed

1 tablespoon hummus

Pinch of salt

4 slices cucumber

2 slices tomato

2 tablespoons shredded carrot

1 clementine, peeled

Directions

Spread one slice of bread with avocado and the other with hummus. Sprinkle with salt. Fill the sandwich with cucumber, tomato and carrot. Slice in half and serve with clementine on the side.

Teriyaki Tofu Rice Bowls

Ingredients

2 (10 ounce) package cooked wild rice blend

1 tablespoon extra-virgin olive oil

1 (18 ounce) package fresh Asian stir-fry vegetables

3 tablespoons teriyaki sauce

1 (7 ounce) package teriyaki-flavor baked tofu, cubed

Directions

1. Prepare rice according to package directions. Transfer the rice from the pouches to a shallow bowl to cool.

2. Heat oil in a medium nonstick skillet over medium heat. Add vegetables and sauté until crisp-tender, 4 to 5 minutes. Add teriyaki sauce; toss well to coat the vegetables. Remove from heat; set aside.

3. Divide the cooled rice among 4 single-serving containers. Top each with one-fourth of the vegetables. Divide tofu among the containers. Seal and refrigerate for up to 4 days. Vent the container and microwave until steaming before serving.

Chopped Salad with Sriracha Tofu & Peanut Dressing

Ingredients

1 (10 ounce) package kale, Brussels sprout, broccoli and cabbage salad mix

1 (12 ounce) package frozen shelled edamame, thawed

2 (7 ounce) packages Sriracha-flavored baked tofu, cubed

1/2 cup spicy peanut vinaigrette

Directions

1. Divide salad mix among 4 single-serving containers with lids. Top each with 1/2 cup edamame and one-fourth of the tofu.
2. Transfer 2 tablespoons vinaigrette into each of 4 small lidded containers and refrigerate for up to 4 days.

3. Seal the salad containers and refrigerate for up to 4 days. Dress with vinaigrette up to 1 day before serving.

Quick Shrimp Puttanesca

Ingredients

8 ounces refrigerated fresh linguine noodles, preferably whole-wheat

1 tablespoon extra-virgin olive oil

1 pound peeled and deveined large shrimp

1 (15 ounce) can no-salt-added tomato sauce

1 ¼ cups frozen quartered artichoke hearts, thawed (8 ounces)

¼ cup chopped pitted Kalamata olives

1 tablespoon capers, rinsed

¼ teaspoon salt

Directions

1. Bring a large pot of water to a boil. Cook linguine according to package instructions. Drain.

2. Meanwhile, heat oil in a large skillet over high heat. Add shrimp in a single layer and cook, undisturbed, until browned on the bottom, 2 to 3 minutes. Stir in tomato sauce. Add artichoke hearts, olives, capers and salt; cook, stirring often, until the shrimp is cooked through and the artichoke hearts are hot, 2 to 3 minutes longer.

3. Add the drained noodles to the sauce and stir to combine. Divide among 4 pasta bowls. Serve hot.

Strawberry & Tuna Spinach Salad

Ingredients

4 cups baby spinach

⅓ cup tuna salad

½ cup sliced white mushrooms

½ cup strawberries

¼ cup sliced red onion

2 tablespoons chopped celery

1 ½ tablespoons slivered almonds

1 tablespoon lemon juice

¼ cup mixed fresh fruit

¼ cup yogurt

Directions

1. Mix spinach, tuna salad, mushrooms, strawberries, and celery in a medium bowl. Drizzle lemon juice and sprinkle almonds on top.
2. Mix fruit and yogurt in a small bowl. Serve on the side.

Quinoa Chickpea Salad with Roasted Red Pepper Hummus Dressing

Ingredients

2 tablespoons hummus, original or roasted red pepper flavor

1 tablespoon lemon juice

1 tablespoon chopped roasted red pepper

2 cups mixed salad greens

½ cup cooked quinoa

½ cup chickpeas, rinsed

1 tablespoon unsalted sunflower seeds

1 tablespoon chopped fresh parsley

Pinch of salt

Pinch of ground pepper

Directions

Stir hummus, lemon juice and red peppers in a small dish. Thin with water to desired consistency for dressing.

Arrange greens, quinoa and chickpeas in a large bowl. Top with sunflower seeds, parsley, salt and pepper. Serve with the dressing.

BBQ Chicken Bowls

Ingredients

8 ounces Yukon Gold potatoes, cut into 1/2-in. pieces

1 tablespoon canola oil

⅞ teaspoon kosher salt, divided

½ teaspoon black pepper, divided

1 ½ tablespoons mayonnaise

1 tablespoon apple cider vinegar

½ teaspoon granulated sugar

2 cups angel hair coleslaw

2 (15 ounce) cans no-salt-added pinto beans, drained

2 cups shredded cooked chicken

6 tablespoons spicy barbecue sauce

½ cup water

½ cup fresh yellow corn kernels

1 tablespoon chopped fresh chives

Directions

Preheat oven to 450 degrees F. Toss potatoes with oil and 1/4 teaspoon each salt and pepper. Spread on a rimmed baking sheet; roast until golden, about 15 minutes.

Whisk together mayonnaise, vinegar, sugar, 1/4 teaspoon salt, and 1/4 teaspoon pepper in a bowl. Add slaw, and toss to coat.

Combine beans, chicken, barbecue sauce, water, and 3/8 teaspoon salt in a saucepan; bring to a simmer over medium-high. Remove from heat; divide among 4 bowls. Top with potatoes, slaw, corn, and chives.

Green Goddess Salad with Chickpeas

Ingredients

Dressing

1 avocado, peeled and pitted

1 ½ cups buttermilk

¼ cup chopped fresh herbs, such as tarragon, sorrel, mint, parsley and/or cilantro

2 tablespoons rice vinegar

½ teaspoon salt

Salad

3 cups chopped romaine lettuce

1 cup sliced cucumber

1 (15 ounce) can chickpeas, rinsed

¼ cup diced low-fat Swiss cheese

6 cherry tomatoes, halved if desired

Directions

To prepare dressing: Place avocado, buttermilk, herbs, vinegar and salt in a blender. Puree until smooth.

To prepare salad: Toss lettuce and cucumber in a bowl with 1/4 cup of the dressing. Top with chickpeas, cheese and tomatoes. (Refrigerate the extra dressing for up to 3 days.)

RECIPES FOR DINNER ON THE ANTI-INFLAMMATORY SJÖGREN DIET

Turkey chilli

Ingredients

1 tbsp rapeseed oil

500g turkey thigh mince (7% fat)

2 large garlic cloves, finely grated

1 chilli, deseeded and chopped

½ tsp dried oregano

2 tsp ground coriander

1 tsp ground cumin

1 tbsp smoked paprika

500g carton passata

2 x 400g cans red kidney beans drained (liquid reserved)

2 tsp vegetable bouillon powder

2 red peppers, deseeded and diced

4 small sweet potatoes (about 140g each)

2 avocados

1 lime, juiced

Directions

STEP 1

Heat the oil in a large pan over a medium heat, then tip in the mince and break it up using a wooden spoon. Stir in the garlic and chilli, and cook for 10 mins until the mince is cooked through. Add the herbs and spices, and cook for a minute more.

STEP 2

Pour in the passata, the reserved liquid from the beans, the bouillon powder and peppers. Cover and cook for 15-20 mins until slightly thickened. Tip in the beans and cook for 3-5 mins more.

STEP 3

Meanwhile, prick two of the sweet potatoes all over using a fork, then microwave on high for 7-10 mins until tender. Mash one of the avocados with half the lime juice in a small bowl.

STEP 4

To serve, halve the potatoes and spoon over half the chilli, then finish with the mashed avocado. Chill the remainder for another day. The chilli will keep covered and chilled for four days or frozen for three months. Reheat in a microwave or pan over low heat until piping hot. Serve with the remaining sweet potatoes and mashed avocado and lime juice, as described above.

Chicken gyros

Ingredients

12 boneless, skinless chicken thighs

Chicken gyros marinade

500g Greek yogurt

2 lemons, juiced, ½ lemon zested

100ml olive oil

4 garlic cloves, very finely grated or crushed

1 tbsp ground coriander

1 tbsp ground cumin

1 tbsp sweet paprika

1 tsp dried oregano

1 tsp dried thyme

1 tsp cayenne pepper

1 tsp crushed black pepper

½ tsp ground cinnamon

To serve

2 red onions, halved and finely sliced

4 tomatoes (plum work well) halved and sliced

Directions

STEP 1

First, whisk all the marinade Ingredients together with 1 tsp salt in a large bowl or, better still, a large plastic container that has a lid. Open out each chicken thigh, cover with a piece of baking parchment and flatten it with your hand, then lift off the paper and cut the thigh in half. Tip into the marinade and mix so it's completely coated. Cover, chill and marinate for at least 1 hr or up to 24 hrs – the longer, the better.

STEP 2

Thread all the chicken onto two skewers so that both skewers go through each piece of meat, packing down tightly as you go to make a compact kebab (see tip, below).

STEP 3

Light a lidded barbecue, and let the flames die down. Once the coals have turned ashen, pile them up on one side with a single layer of coals scattered around the other side. Lay the chicken kebab on the side of the barbecue with only a few coals underneath. Put the lid down and cook for 45 mins, turning every 15 mins. To finish, lift the lid and roll the kebab over to the hotter side to char the meat, turning it every few minutes until well browned and cooked through. Prise the chicken pieces apart in the centre to check they're cooked, or use a digital cooking thermometer – it should read 70C or more. Leave to rest for 5-10 mins while you cook the pittas (see recipe, opposite). Bring the kebab to the table and carve into thin slices with a serrated knife. Pile the carved meat into the warm pittas, then the sliced red onions and tomatoes, chips and tzatziki

Fish pie with pea & dill mash

Ingredients

375g potatoes, cut into chunks

175g leeks, thickly sliced

160g frozen peas

2 tbsp half-fat crème fraîche

½ lemon, zested and juiced

2 tbsp chopped fresh dill

½ tsp vegetable bouillon powder

100g cherry tomatoes, halved

250g skinless cod loin, cut into large chunks

50g Atlantic prawns (thawed if frozen)

veg, to serve (optional)

Directions

STEP 1

Heat oven to 200C/180C fan/gas 6. Cook the potatoes in a pan of boiling water for 10 mins, with the leeks in a covered steamer over the pan. Remove the steamer, add the peas to the potatoes and cook for 10 mins more. Drain the peas and potatoes, then mash with ½ tbsp crème fraîche, the lemon zest and juice, dill and bouillon.

STEP 2

Arrange the leeks in a shallow ovenproof pie dish (about 18 x 24cm). Add the tomatoes, cod and prawns, then dot over the rest of the crème fraîche. Spoon over the mash, then spread it lightly to the edges with a fork.

STEP 3

Bake for 30-35 mins until bubbling round the sides of the dish. Serve with veg, if you like. If you make this ahead and are cooking from cold, bake for about 10 mins longer.

Wild mushroom & ricotta rice with rosemary & thyme

Ingredients

15g dried porcini mushrooms

1 tbsp balsamic vinegar

1 tbsp vegetable bouillon powder

1 tbsp rapeseed oil

1 large onion, finely chopped

200g pack small button mushrooms

1 tbsp fresh thyme leaves

1 tsp chopped rosemary

3 garlic cloves, sliced

170g brown basmati rice

2 leeks, washed and sliced

50g ricotta

15g vegetarian Italian-style hard cheese, finely grated

parsley, to serve

Directions

STEP 1

Put the dried mushrooms in a measuring jug and pour over 800ml boiling water. Stir in the balsamic and bouillon. Leave to soak.

STEP 2

Heat the oil in a large wok or frying pan and fry the onion for 8 mins until soft and golden. Add the button mushrooms, thyme, rosemary, garlic and black pepper, then cook, stirring occasionally, for 5 mins. Pour in the dried mushrooms and liquid, then stir in the rice and leeks.

STEP 3

Cover and leave to simmer for 30 mins until the liquid has been absorbed and the rice is tender but still nutty. Remove from the heat, then stir in the ricotta and grated cheese, and serve scattered with parsley leaves.

Chilli chicken & peanut pies

Ingredients

For the mash

500g potatoes, peeled and chopped

2 x 400g cans cannellini beans, drained

3 tbsp chopped fresh coriander

1 tsp chilli powder

For the chicken filling

2 tsp olive oil

2 tbsp finely chopped ginger

1 red chilli, deseeded for less spice

2 tbsp cumin seeds

2 tbsp ground coriander

1 tsp chilli powder

400g leeks, thickly sliced

1 red pepper, deseeded and diced

1 green pepper, deseeded and diced

2 large skinless chicken breasts, about 400g, diced

400g can chopped tomatoes

2 tbsp tomato purée

2 tsp vegetable bouillon

3 tbsp peanut butter (with no sugar or palm oil)

320g broccoli, to serve

Directions

STEP 1

Heat oven to 200C/180C fan/gas 6. Cook the potatoes in a steamer for 15 mins until tender. Meanwhile, start the chicken filling. Heat the oil in a non-stick pan, add the ginger and chilli, and stir over a medium heat until starting to soften. Stir in the dried spices, leeks and peppers. Cook, stirring frequently, until softened.

STEP 2

Add the chicken and stir-fry until it begins to colour, then tip in the tomatoes, squeeze in some tomato purée and add the bouillon and 150ml water. Cover and simmer for 10 mins.

STEP 3

Mix the peanut butter with 100ml water, then stir into the stew and cook for 5 mins more. Spoon the mixture equally into two 24 x 18cm shallow pie dishes.

STEP 4

For the mash, tip the beans into a bowl, add the coriander and chilli powder and mash well. Add the steamed potatoes and roughly mash into the beans so it still has a little texture. Pile on top of the filling in the pie dishes and carefully spread over the filling to enclose it. Bake one of the pies for 35 mins.

STEP 5

Meanwhile, cook half of the broccoli and serve with the pie. Chill the other pie with the remaining broccoli for another day. Will keep chilled for up to three days. Reheat the remaining pie as above, adding an extra 15 mins to the cooking time.

One-pot harissa chicken

Ingredients

4 skinless chicken breasts

1 tsp ground cumin

1 tbsp olive oil

1 onion, finely sliced

400g can cherry tomato

2 tbsp harissa paste (we used Belazu Rose Harissa)

1 tbsp clear honey

2 medium courgettes, thickly sliced

400g can chickpea, drained and rinsed

Directions

STEP 1

Season the chicken breasts all over with the cumin and lots of ground black pepper. Heat the oil in a large non-stick frying pan and cook the chicken with the onion for 4 mins. Turn the chicken over and cook for a further 3 mins. Stir the onions around the chicken regularly as they cook.

STEP 2

Tip the tomatoes and 250ml water into the pan and stir in the harissa, honey, courgettes and chickpeas. Bring to a gentle simmer and cook for 15 mins until the chicken is tender and the sauce has thickened slightly.

Crispy za'atar chicken pilaf with pomegranate

Ingredients

8 skin-on chicken thighs

3 tbsp olive oil

2 garlic cloves, crushed

1 lemon, juiced

3 tbsp za'atar

70g pomegranate seeds

½ small bunch of parsley, finely chopped

For the rice

1 tbsp olive oil

50g butter

2 large onions, sliced

220g basmati rice

350ml hot chicken stock

70g pistachios, chopped

1 tsp chilli flakes

Directions

STEP 1

Toss together the chicken thighs oil, 1 tsp salt, garlic and lemon juice in a large bowl. Cover and chill for at least 1 hr, or up to 12 hrs.

STEP 2

Heat the oven to 180C/160C fan/gas 4, and heat a frying pan over a high heat. Fry the chicken, skin-side down, for 5-7 mins, or until golden and crisp. Transfer to a baking tray and sprinkle with the za'atar, then roast for 10 mins.

STEP 3

For the rice, heat the oil and butter in a large, shallow casserole or frying pan over a low-medium heat. Fry the onions with a pinch of salt for 15 mins until caramelised and sticky. Stir in the rice, stock, pistachios and chilli flakes. Season. Arrange the roasted chicken thighs on top of the rice, and pour over any roasting juices from the tray. Cook in the oven for 45 mins, or until the rice is tender. Remove from the oven, cover and rest for 5 mins.

STEP 4

Scatter the chicken pilaf with the pomegranate seeds and parsley, then serve in shallow bowls.

Pork with cucumber & apricot couscous

Ingredients

30g fresh coriander

4 small garlic cloves, chopped

2 tsp sumac

1 tbsp olive oil

400g pork fillet

1½ tsp smoked paprika

For the couscous

drop of olive oil, for roasting

2 red onions, halved and sliced

1 aubergine, cut into 1cm cubes

200g wholemeal giant couscous

small bunch of spring onions (about 100g), sliced

½ large cucumber (about 320g), chopped

1 lemon, zested plus 2 tbsp juice

2 tbsp extra virgin olive oil

15g mint, leaves chopped

8 fresh apricots (about 320g)

25g toasted flaked almonds

Directions

STEP 1

Heat the oven to 190C/170C fan/gas 5. Put the coriander in a small bowl with the garlic, sumac, oil and 2 tbsp water, then blitz using a hand blender until smooth. Rub a quarter of it all over the pork, then put the pork on a large baking tray and sprinkle over the paprika.

STEP 2

For the couscous, rub a drop of oil over the red onions and aubergine, then scatter around the pork. (If your tray isn't large enough, use two.)

Roast for 25 mins. Check the pork and if it isn't cooked but the vegetables are, take the vegetables out of the oven and cook the pork for another 10-15 mins until the juices run clear.

Healthy roast dinner

Ingredients

285g medium potatoes, thickly sliced

4 small carrots (160g), halved lengthways

2 x 80g red onions, cut into quarters

170g large Brussels sprouts (about 8-10), trimmed

2½ tsp rapeseed oil

2 tsp thyme leaves

2 tsp balsamic vinegar

1 large garlic clove, finely grated

2 pinches of English mustard powder

170g thick, lean fillet steak

½ tsp vegetable bouillon powder

Directions

STEP 1

Heat the oven to 180C/160C fan/gas 4. Bring a large pan of water to the boil and cook the potatoes for 5 mins. Drain, reserving the water.

STEP 2

Toss the potatoes, carrots, onions and sprouts with 2 tsp of the oil to coat. Arrange on a non-stick baking sheet, spaced apart. Scatter with 1 tsp of the thyme, grind over some black pepper, then roast for 30 mins.

STEP 3

Meanwhile, mix 1 tsp of the vinegar with the garlic, remaining thyme and oil, the mustard and plenty of black pepper. Rub this over the steak, put in a shallow dish and set aside. Mix the rest of the vinegar with the bouillon and 125ml of the reserved water from step 1, then set aside. After 30 mins, turn the veg over and roast for 15 mins more.

STEP 4

Meanwhile, heat a small non-stick frying pan over a medium-high heat. Lift the steak out of the marinade, shake off the excess and fry for 2-3 mins on each side until cooked to your liking. Remove to a board and leave to rest. Pour the leftover marinade into the frying pan and bubble until thickened slightly to make a gravy. Slice the steak and serve with the roast veg and gravy on the side.

Beef bourguignon

Ingredients

1.6kg braising steak, cut into large chunks

3 bay leaves

small bunch thyme

2 bottles cheap red wine

2 tbsp oil

3 large or 6 normal carrots, cut into large chunks

2 onions, roughly chopped

3 tbsp plain flour

1 tbsp tomato purée

To serve

small knob butter

300g bacon lardons

500g pearl onions or small shallots, peeled

400g mushrooms, halved

chopped parsley

Directions

STEP 1

Tip 1.6kg braising steak, cut into large chunks, into a large bowl with 3 bay leaves, a small bunch of thyme, 2 bottles of red wine and some pepper, then cover and leave in the fridge overnight.

STEP 2

Heat the oven to 200C/180C fan/gas 6.

STEP 3

Place a colander over another large bowl and strain the marinated meat, keeping the wine.

STEP 4

Heat 1 tbsp oil in a large frying pan, then brown the meat in batches, transferring to a plate once browned. When all the meat is browned, pour a little wine into the now-empty frying pan and bubble to release any caramelised bits from the pan.

STEP 5

Heat 1 tbsp oil in a large casserole and fry 3 large or 6 normal carrots, cut into large chunks, and 2 roughly chopped onions until they start to colour.

Stir in 3 tbsp plain flour for 1 min, then add 1 tbsp tomato purée.

STEP 6

Add the beef and any juices, the wine from the frying pan and the rest of the wine and herbs. Season and bring to a simmer. Give everything a good stir, then cover.

STEP 7

Transfer to the oven and bake for 2 hrs until the meat is really tender. Cool. Will freeze for up to 3 months.

STEP 8

To serve, defrost completely overnight in the fridge if frozen, then place on a low heat to warm through.

STEP 9

Meanwhile, heat a small knob of butter in a frying pan and add 300g bacon lardons and 500g peeled pearl onions or small shallots. Sizzle for about 10 mins until the bacon starts to crisp and the onions soften and colour.

STEP 10

Add 400g halved mushrooms and fry for another 5 mins, then stir everything into the stew and heat for 10 mins more. Serve scattered with chopped parsley.

Stuffed mushrooms

Ingredients

4-6 medium-large portobello mushrooms

125g unsmoked bacon lardons

1 shallot, finely chopped

1 garlic clove, finely chopped

4 tbsp dried breadcrumbs

1 tsp dried sage

50g medium cheddar, grated

Directions

STEP 1

Heat oven to 220C/200C fan/gas 7. Wipe the mushrooms to remove any dirt, then turn upside down and remove the stalks. Place on a baking tray top-side down.

STEP 2

Fry the lardons for 8-10 mins until just starting to crisp up, then finely chop the shallot, mushroom stalks and garlic. Add to the bacon and fry on a moderate heat for about 5 mins until all the Ingredients are cooked.

STEP 3

Take off the heat and add the breadcrumbs and sage, then stir to make an even mixture. Spoon into the hollows of the mushrooms and sprinkle with the grated cheese.

STEP 4

Bake for approximately 8-10 mins until the cheese has melted. Serve with crusty bread and a green salad.

Balsamic beef with beetroot & rocket

Ingredients

240g beef sirloin, fat trimmed

1 tbsp balsamic vinegar

2 tsp thyme leaves

2 garlic cloves, 1 finely grated, 1 sliced

2 tsp rapeseed oil

2 red onions, halved and sliced

175g fine beans, trimmed

2 cooked beetroot, halved and cut into wedges

6 pitted Kalamata olives, quartered

2 handfuls rocket

Directions

STEP 1

Beat the steak with a rolling pin until it is about the thickness of two £1 coins, then cut into two equal pieces. In a bowl, mix the balsamic, thyme, grated garlic, half the oil and a grinding of black pepper. Place the steaks in the marinade and set aside.

STEP 2

Heat the remaining 1 tsp oil in a large non-stick frying pan, and fry the onions and garlic for 8-10 mins, stirring frequently, until soft and starting to brown. Meanwhile, steam the beans for 4-6 mins or until just tender.

STEP 3

Push the onion mixture to one side in the pan. Lift the steaks from the bowl, shake off any excess marinade, and sear in the pan for 2½-3 mins, turning once, until cooked but still a little pink inside. Pile the beans onto plates and place the steaks on top. Add the beetroot wedges, olives and remaining marinade to the pan and cook briefly to heat through, then spoon on top and around the steaks. Add the rocket and serve.

Spinach omelette

Ingredients

85g wholewheat penne

frozen spinach, once thawed and squeezed it should be around 185-200g, roughly chopped

3 garlic cloves, finely grated

1 tsp smoked paprika, plus an extra pinch to serve

6 pitted green olives, sliced into rings

4 eggs

145g can tuna in spring water, drained

1 tsp rapeseed oil

For the salad

1 red onion, halved and thinly sliced

½ lemon, juiced

2 tomatoes, cut into thin wedges

20g feta

a few thyme leaves, to serve (optional)

Directions

STEP 1

First, for the salad, put the red onion and lemon juice in a bowl and scrunch together using your hands. Set aside for the onions to soften.

STEP 2

Meanwhile boil the penne for 12 mins, or following pack instructions, until tender. Drain and cool under running cold water, then drain again thoroughly. Tip into a bowl and mix with the spinach, garlic, paprika, olives and eggs. Fold in the tuna.

STEP 3

Heat the oil in a 20cm non-stick frying pan. Tip in the spinach and egg mixture, then cook covered over a gentle heat for about 10 mins until set. Turn out onto a plate and slide back into the pan to cook the other side for 5 mins. Serve topped with the red onions, tomatoes and crumbled feta, and sprinkle with a little extra paprika and thyme, if you like. Cut into wedges to serve.

Tagliatelle with vegetable ragu

Ingredients

1 onion, finely chopped

2 celery sticks, finely chopped

2 carrots, diced

4 garlic cloves, crushed

1 tbsp each tomato purée and balsamic vinegar

250g diced vegetables, such as courgettes, peppers and mushroom

50g red lentil

2 x 400g cans chopped tomatoes with basil

250g tagliatelle (or your favourite pasta)

2 tbsp shaved parmesan (optional)

Directions

STEP 1

Tip the onion, celery and carrots into a large non-stick saucepan and add 2-3 tbsp water or stock, if you have some. Cook gently, stirring often, until the vegetables are soft.

STEP 2

Add the garlic, tomato purée and balsamic vinegar, cook on a high heat for 1 min more, add the diced veg, lentils, tomatoes, then bring up to the boil.

STEP 3

Turn to a simmer, then cook for about 20 mins. Meanwhile, cook the pasta following pack instructions, then drain. Season the ragu and serve with pasta and Parmesan on top, if you like.

Hummus flatbread pizzas with roasted veg

Ingredients

1 courgette (about 200g), sliced into rounds (or use frozen grilled Mediterranean vegetables)

1 large red pepper, halved, deseeded and cut into 8 wedges

½ tbsp olive oil

pinch of dried oregano

100g hummus

3 pitted Kalamata olives, quartered

small handful of basil leaves

extra virgin olive oil, for drizzling

For the flatbreads

100g spelt wholemeal flour, plus extra for dusting

1 tsp baking powder

100g natural bio yogurt

Directions

STEP 1

Heat the oven to 220C/200C fan/gas 7. Toss the courgettes and peppers with the olive oil on a baking sheet. Sprinkle over the oregano and some black pepper. Roast for 30-35 mins, turning the veg halfway through, until softened and starting to char.

STEP 2

Meanwhile, make the flatbreads. Tip the flour into a bowl and stir in the baking powder. Stir in the yogurt using a cutlery knife until you have a soft, slightly wet dough. Cut the dough in half and set aside to rest for 10 mins.

STEP 3

Heat a large non-stick dry frying pan over a low heat. Knead one of the dough halves briefly on a well-floured work surface until it's smooth and elastic, then roll out into a roughly 17cm circle. Put the flatbread in the pan and cook for 3 mins, then flip and cook for 3 mins more until cooked through. Transfer to a serving plate. Repeat with the second dough half.

STEP 4

Spread the hummus over the flatbreads, then pile on the roasted veg and scatter over the olives and basil. Drizzle over a little extra virgin olive oil and serve warm.

RECIPES FOR SIDE DISH ON THE ANTI-INFLAMMATORY SJÖGREN DIET

Simple sourdough

Ingredients

For the starter

700g strong white flour

For the loaf

500g strong white flour, plus extra for dusting

1 tsp fine salt

1 tbsp clear honey

300g sourdough starter

flavourless oil, for greasing

Instructions

STEP 1

First, make your starter. In a large bowl, mix together 100g of the flour with 125ml slightly warm water. Whisk together until smooth and lump-free.

STEP 2

Transfer the starter to a large jar (a 1-litre Kilner jar is good) or a plastic container. Leave the jar or container lid ajar for 1 hr or so in a warm place (around 25C is ideal), then seal and set aside for 24 hrs.

STEP 3

For the next 6 days, you will need to 'feed' the starter. Each day, tip away half of the original starter, add an extra 100g of flour and 125ml slightly warm water, and stir well. Try to do this at the same time every day.

STEP 4

After 3-4 days you should start to see bubbles appearing on the surface, and it will smell yeasty and a little acidic. This is a good indicator that the starter is working.

STEP 5

On day 7, the starter should be quite bubbly and smell much sweeter. It is now ready to be used in baking.

STEP 6

Tip the flour, 225ml warm water, the salt, honey and the starter into a bowl, or a mixer fitted with a dough hook. Stir with a wooden spoon, or on a slow setting in the machine, until combined – add extra flour if it's too sticky or a little extra warm water if it's too dry.

STEP 7

Tip onto a lightly floured surface and knead for 10 mins until soft and elastic – you should be able to stretch it without it tearing. If you're using a mixer, turn up the speed a little and mix for 5 mins.

STEP 8

Place the dough in a large, well-oiled bowl and cover. Leave in a warm place to rise for 3 hrs. You may not see much movement, but don't be disheartened, as sourdough takes much longer to rise than a conventional yeasted bread.

STEP 9

Line a medium-sized bowl with a clean tea towel and flour it really well or, if you have a proving basket, you can use this (see tips below). Tip the dough back onto your work surface and knead briefly to knock out any air bubbles. Shape the dough into a smooth ball and dust it with flour.

STEP 10

Place the dough, seam-side up, in the bowl or proving basket, cover loosely and leave at room temperature until roughly doubled in size. The time it takes for your bread to rise will vary depending on the strength of your starter and the temperature in the room, anywhere from 4-8 hrs. The best indicators are your eyes, so don't worry too much about timings here. You can also prove your bread overnight in the fridge. Remove it in the morning and let it continue rising for another hour or 2 at room temperature. The slower the rise, the deeper the flavour you will achieve.

STEP 11

Place a large baking tray in the oven, and heat to 230C/210C fan/gas 8. Fill a small roasting tin with a little water and place this in the bottom of the oven to create steam. Remove the baking tray from the oven, sprinkle with flour, then carefully tip the risen dough onto the tray.

STEP 12

Slash the top a few times with a sharp knife, if you like, then bake for 35-40 mins until golden brown. It will sound hollow when tapped on the bottom. Leave to cool on a wire rack for 20 mins before serving.

Avocado panzanella

Ingredients

800g mix of ripe tomatoes

1 garlic clove, crushed

1½ tbsp capers, drained and rinsed

1 ripe avocado, stoned, peeled and chopped

1 small red onion, very thinly sliced

175g ciabatta or crusty loaf

4 tbsp extra virgin olive oil

2 tbsp red wine vinegar

small handful basil leaves

Instructions

STEP 1

Halve or roughly chop the tomatoes (depending on size) and put them in a bowl. Season well and add the garlic, capers, avocado and onion, and mix well. Set aside for 10 mins.

STEP 2

Meanwhile, tear or slice the ciabatta into 3cm chunks and place in a large serving bowl or on a platter. Drizzle with half the olive oil, half the vinegar and add some seasoning. When ready to serve, pour over the tomatoes and any juices. Scatter with the basil leaves and drizzle over the remaining oil and vinegar. Give it a final stir and serve immediately.

Red cabbage with mulled Port & pears

Ingredients

1 large red cabbage, quartered, cored and thinly sliced

1 large onion, sliced

200ml port

1 large cinnamon stick

pinch ground cloves

2 star anise

2 tbsp soft brown sugar

1 tbsp red wine vinegar

4 pears, diced

Instructions

STEP 1

Put all the Ingredients except the pears in a large pan and cover with a tight- fitting lid. Cook on a low heat for 1 hr, then stir through the pears. Cover and cook for 1 hr more until the cabbage is really tender. If at any point the cabbage looks dry, add a splash of water. If there is still liquid in the pan at the end, turn the heat right up to evaporate it. Season with a little salt and serve. The cabbage can be prepared ahead and either chilled or frozen. Then reheat in the pan or in a microwave.

Quick pickled cucumbers

Ingredients

1 large cucumber, ends trimmed, cut in half widthways and spiralized into thick ribbons

1 tsp flaky sea salt

1 tbsp white wine vinegar

1 tbsp caster sugar

½ tsp coriander seeds

a small handful of dill, leaves picked

Instructions

STEP 1

Toss the cucumber ribbons with the salt in a colander. Leave for 15 mins then squeeze out any excess moisture with your hands and pat the ribbons dry with a tea towel.

STEP 2

Mix the other Ingredients together in a small bowl then stir in the cucumber.

Roasted garlic & parmesan sprouts

Ingredients

600g brussels sprouts, halved

50g butter, melted

2 garlic cloves, crushed

50g panko breadcrumbs

25g parmesan or vegetarian alternative, finely grated

Instructions

STEP 1

Heat the oven to 200C/180C fan/gas 6. Tip the brussels sprouts into a bowl, drizzle over the melted butter, add the garlic and season. Toss the sprouts until they're well coated in the butter, then add the breadcrumbs and parmesan, and toss again.

STEP 2

Tip the sprouts onto a baking tray, making sure they're well-spaced apart in a single layer. (If they're packed too closely they will steam instead of roasting.) Place as many as possible cut-side down for maximum crispiness. Press any excess crumbs onto the sprouts to help them stick.

STEP 3

Roast for 25-30 mins until crisp and golden.

Sausage, sage & onion stuffing

Ingredients

2 onions, sliced

25g butter

1 small Bramley apple, peeled, cored and diced

2 x 400g packs meaty Cumberland sausages, removed from their skins

handful sage, leaves chopped, plus extra for topping

140g granary breadcrumbs

Instructions

STEP 1

Fry 2 sliced onions in 25g butter for 5 mins, then add 1 small diced Bramley apple and cook briefly.

STEP 2

Cool, then mix with 800g Cumberland sausages, skins removed, the chopped handful of sage, 140g granary breadcrumbs and seasoning.

STEP 3

Use to stuff the neck end of the bird, then roll any leftovers into balls. Or, pack the whole mixture into a 1kg loaf tin and top with extra sage leaves.

STEP 4

Bake with turkey for 30-40 mins. Drain off any fat and serve sliced.

Homemade vegan bagels

Ingredients

7g sachet dried yeast

4 tbsp sugar

2 tsp salt

450g bread flour

poppy, fennel and/or sesame seeds to sprinkle on top (optional)

Instructions

STEP 1

Tip the yeast and 1 tbsp sugar into a large bowl, and pour over 100ml warm water. Leave for 10 mins until the mixture becomes frothy.

STEP 2

Pour 200ml warm water into the bowl, then stir in the salt and half the flour. Keep adding the remaining flour (you may not have to use it all) and mixing with your hands until you have a soft but not sticky dough. Then knead for 10 mins until the dough feels smooth and elastic. Shape into a ball and put in a clean, lightly oiled bowl. Cover loosely and leave in a warm place until doubled in size, about 1hr.

STEP 3

Heat the oven to 220C/200C fan/gas 7. On a lightly floured surface, divide the dough into 10 pieces, each about 85g. Shape each piece into a flattish ball, then take a wooden spoon and use the handle to make a hole in the middle of each ball. Slip the spoon into the hole, then twirl the bagel around the spoon to make a hole about 3cm wide. Cover the bagel loosely while you shape the remaining dough.

STEP 4

Meanwhile, bring a large pan of water to the boil and tip in the remaining sugar. Slip the bagels into the boiling water – no more than four at a time. Cook for 1-2 mins, turning over in the water until the bagels have puffed slightly and a skin has formed. Remove with a slotted spoon and drain away any excess water. Sprinkle over your choice of topping and place on a baking tray lined with parchment. Bake in the oven for 25 mins until browned and crisp – the bases should sound hollow when tapped. Leave to cool on a wire rack, then serve with your favourite filling.

Cheese-stuffed garlic dough balls with a tomato sauce dip

Ingredients

50g butter, cubed

300g strong white bread flour

7g sachet fast-action dried yeast

1 tbsp caster sugar

200g block mozzarella, cut into 1.5cm cubes

65g gruyère, coarsely grated (optional)

For the garlic butter

100g butter

2 garlic cloves, crushed

1 rosemary sprig, leaves picked and finely chopped

For the tomato sauce dip

1 tbsp olive oil, plus extra for the bowl and baking sheet

1 garlic clove, sliced

250g passata

1 tsp red wine vinegar

1 tsp caster sugar

pinch of chilli flakes

½ small bunch of basil, torn, plus extra to serve

Instructions

STEP 1

Heat 175ml water in a saucepan until steaming, then add the butter. Remove from the heat and leave to cool until the mixture is just warm (it should not be hot). Combine the flour, yeast, sugar and 1 tsp salt in a large bowl or stand mixer. Add the cooled butter mixture, and mix to a soft dough using a wooden spoon or the mixer. Knead for 10 mins by hand (or 5 mins using a mixer) until the dough feels bouncy and smooth. Transfer to an oiled bowl and cover with a clean tea towel. Leave somewhere warm to rise for 1½-2 hrs, or until doubled in size. Alternatively, leave to prove in the fridge overnight.

STEP 2

Oil and line a baking sheet with baking parchment. Knock the air out of the dough, then knead again for several minutes. Flatten a small piece of dough (about 20g) into a disc, and put a cube of the mozzarella and a pinch of the gruyère into the middle of the disc. Enclose the cheeses with the dough, then roll into a ball. Transfer to the prepared baking sheet. Repeat with the remaining cheese and dough, placing the dough balls ½cm apart on the baking sheet – they should be just touching after proving. Cover with a clean tea towel and leave somewhere warm to rise for 30 mins.

STEP 3

Meanwhile, make the garlic butter. Melt the butter in a small pan over a low heat, then stir in the garlic and rosemary. Remove from the heat and set aside until needed. Heat the oven to 180C/160C fan/gas 4. Brush the risen dough balls with the garlic butter, then bake for 25-30 mins until the dough balls are cooked through and the middles are oozing.

STEP 4

While the dough balls are baking, make the tomato sauce dip. Heat the oil in a saucepan and fry the garlic for 30 seconds. Tip in the passata, vinegar, sugar and chilli flakes, and simmer for 10 mins until thickened. Season to taste and stir in the basil. Brush the warm dough balls with any remaining garlic butter, then serve with the tomato sauce dip on the side for dunking.

Sticky spiced red cabbage

Ingredients

1 tbsp olive oil

1 medium-size red cabbage, quartered, cored and shredded

1 finger-size piece fresh root ginger, finely chopped

2 onions, sliced

1 tsp ground allspice

1 tbsp mustard seed

100g golden caster sugar

150ml red wine vinegar

Instructions

STEP 1

Heat oil in a large saucepan, add cabbage, ginger, onions, allspice and mustard seeds, then cook for 5 mins until just starting to wilt.

STEP 2

Scatter over the sugar and pour in the vinegar. Cover pan, gently cook for 10 mins, then remove lid and turn up the heat to medium. Simmer the liquid in the cabbage for about 20 mins, stirring occasionally, then stir continuously for the last few mins until all the liquid has evaporated and becomes sticky on the bottom of the pan. Tip cabbage into a large bowl and serve.

Rye sourdough bread

Ingredients

For the starter

250g wholemeal rye flour

For the bread

100g active rye starter (see above)

500g wholemeal rye flour, extra for dusting

10g fine salt

25g butter, softened, for the tin

Instructions

STEP 1

Day 1: To begin your starter, mix 50g of the flour with 50g tepid water in a jar or, better still, a plastic container. Make sure all the flour is incorporated and leave, covered with a tea towel, at room temperature for 24 hrs.

STEP 2

Days 2, 3, 4 & 5 : Mix 25g flour with 25g tepid water and stir into yesterday's mixture. Make sure all the flour is incorporated and leave, covered with a tea towel, at room temperature for 24 hrs.

STEP 3

Day 6: The mix should be really bubbly and giving off a strong smell of alcohol. A teaspoonful of the starter should float in warm water if ready. If not, continue adding 25g flour and 25g tepid water into the mixture daily until it becomes active.

If your jar is becoming full, spoon half the mix out of the jar and continue. You now have rye starter, which is a malty flavoured base to sourdough bread. Keep it in the fridge (it will stay dormant) and 12 hrs before you want to use it, spoon half of it off and feed it with 100g flour and 100g water. Leave, covered, at room temperature.

STEP 4

Tip 100g of the starter into a bowl and add 400g of tepid water. Whisk or rub the two together with your hands, don't worry if there are a few lumps. Add the flour and bring together (with a spatula or your hand) into a thick, sticky dough, making sure all the flour is mixed in, including any dry bits on the sides of the bowl. Cover with a damp tea towel and leave at room temperature for 2 hrs.

STEP 5

Work the salt into the dough then leave, covered, for another 2 hrs.

STEP 6

Heavily butter a 900g loaf tin. Dust the work surface with more rye flour, then scrape all the dough out. Mould the dough into a block roughly the same size as the tin and sit it in the tin. Press the dough down so it fills it completely and scatter the top generously with more flour. Leave the loaf out, uncovered, for 2 hrs until it's risen by about a quarter and gone craggy on the top, or leave it in the fridge, uncovered, overnight. This will give it an even deeper flavour.

STEP 7

Heat the oven to 230/210C fan/gas 8 with a shelf in the middle of the oven and a shelf below with a roasting tray on it. Put the loaf on the middle tray and carefully pour a small glass of water into the roasting tray. Cook for 50-55 mins until hollow sounding when tapped. (The middle of the loaf will read 98C on a digital thermometer when ready.) Remove the tin and leave to cool on a wire rack for at least 4 hrs. Will keep for 3-4 days in an airtight container.

Carrot & sugar snap salad

Ingredients

1 tbsp hoisin sauce

juice ½ lime

2cm/¾in fresh ginger, peeled and grated

200g sugar snap peas, thinly sliced

3 carrots, coarsely grated

½ small bunch coriander, roughly chopped

Instructions

STEP 1

Make the dressing by whisking the hoisin, lime juice and ginger with 2 tbsp cold water.

STEP 2

In a large bowl, mix the sugar snap peas, carrots and coriander. Pour over the dressing and mix to coat.

Sriracha & lime potato salad

Ingredients

750g new potatoes, halved if large

80g mayonnaise

50g soured cream

2 tbsp sriracha

1 lime, zested and juiced

1 tsp honey

6 spring onions, finely sliced

½ small bunch of coriander, finely chopped

½ tsp chilli flakes (optional)

Instructions

STEP 1

Tip the potatoes into a large pan of cold salted water. Bring to the boil, then reduce the heat and simmer for 15-18 mins until tender. Drain and leave to cool completely.

STEP 2

Whisk the mayonnaise with the soured cream, sriracha, lime zest and juice, the honey, half the spring onions, most of the coriander and some seasoning.

STEP 3

Toss the cooled potatoes with the sriracha-mayonnaise mixture until all the potatoes are coated. Tip into a serving bowl and scatter over the remaining spring onions, the rest of the coriander and chilli flakes, if you like.

Classic coleslaw

Ingredients

6 carrots, peeled

1 small white cabbage

large pinch, golden caster sugar

3 tbsp cider vinegar

1 tbsp mustard (any you've got)

200g mayonnaise

1 red apple, cut into matchsticks (optional)

100g cheddar, grated (optional)

Instructions

STEP 1

Coarsely grate the carrot and finely shred the cabbage (use a food processor with a grating/slicing blade or do it by hand) and tip into a bowl. Season with salt, then add the sugar and vinegar and toss everything together. Leave for 20 mins for the vegetables to very lightly pickle.

STEP 2

Stir through the mustard and mayonnaise and add any other bits you want to, then serve. Can be made a day ahead and chilled.

Honey-roasted parsnips

Ingredients

500g parsnips

1 tbsp flour

1 tbsp honey

2 tbsp sunflower oil

2 tbsp butter

Instructions

STEP 1

Top and tail 500g parsnips, cutting any larger ones in half lengthways, then put in a large saucepan, cover with salted water, bring to the boil and cook for 5 mins.

STEP 2

Drain in a colander and let them steam-dry for a few mins.

STEP 3

Heat oven to 190C/170C fan/ gas 5.

STEP 4

Sprinkle 1 tbsp flour and 1 tbsp honey over the parsnips and toss to coat.

STEP 5

Put the parsnips in a roasting tin with 2 tbsp sunflower oil, 2 tbsp butter and seasoning.

STEP 6

Roast for 40 mins, turning halfway, until golden.

PART 5: LIFESTYLE STRATEGIES FOR TREATMENT EFFECTIVENESS

Managing Sjögren's syndrome involves more than just medical treatment—it's about adopting lifestyle strategies that can really make a difference in how you feel day to day. Here are some practical tips to help you manage symptoms and enhance your overall well-being:

1. **Stay Hydrated**: Keep yourself well-hydrated by drinking plenty of water throughout the day. Using a humidifier in your home can also help with dryness, especially for your eyes and mouth.

2. **Eye Care**: Use artificial tears or eye drops regularly to keep your eyes moist. Try to avoid dry

or windy environments that can worsen dry eye symptoms.

3. **Oral Hygiene**: Take good care of your teeth by brushing regularly with fluoride toothpaste. Using mouthwashes or saliva substitutes can help with dry mouth. Don't forget to see your dentist regularly to prevent dental issues.

4. **Healthy Eating**: Aim for a balanced diet that includes plenty of fruits, vegetables, and foods rich in omega-3 fatty acids like fish or flaxseeds. This can help reduce inflammation and support your overall health.

5. **Joint Health**: Stay active with gentle exercises like stretching, walking, or swimming to keep your joints flexible and minimize stiffness. Physical

therapy might also be beneficial for managing joint pain.

6. **Manage Fatigue**: Get enough rest and establish a regular sleep routine to combat fatigue. Relaxation techniques such as deep breathing or meditation can also help you unwind and recharge.

7. **Avoid Smoking and Limit Alcohol**: Both smoking and excessive alcohol can worsen symptoms of Sjögren's syndrome. Quitting smoking and moderating alcohol intake can improve your overall health and symptom management.

8. **Protect Yourself**: Practice good hygiene to reduce the risk of infections, especially handwashing. Stay up to date with vaccinations as recommended by your doctor to protect your immune system.

9. **Emotional Support**: Living with a chronic illness can be challenging emotionally. Seek support from loved ones, consider joining support groups, or talk to a therapist for additional support and coping strategies.

10. **Regular Check-ups**: Stay in touch with your healthcare team and attend regular check-ups. This allows your doctor to monitor your condition and adjust your treatment plan as needed.

Incorporating these lifestyle tips into your daily routine can complement medical treatments and improve your quality of life with Sjögren's syndrome. Remember to always consult with your healthcare provider before making any changes to your treatment plan or lifestyle.